Health Measurement Scales

A Practical Guide to Their Development and Use

Second Edition

David L. Streiner

and

Geoffrey R. Norman

Department of Clinical Epidemiology and Biostatistics,
McMaster University, Hamilton, Ontario, Canada

OXFORD · NEW YORK · TOKYO
OXFORD UNIVERSITY PRESS

Oxford University Press, Walton Street, Oxford OX2 6DP
Oxford New York
Athens Auckland Bangkok Bombay
Calcutta Cape Town Dar es Salaam Delhi
Florence Hong Kong Istanbul Karachi
Kuala Lumpur Madras Madrid Melbourne
Mexico City Nairobi Paris Singapore
Taipei Tokyo Toronto
and associated companies in
Berlin Ibadan

Oxford is a trade mark of Oxford University Press

Published in the United States
by Oxford University Press Inc., New York

First edition published 1989
Second edition published 1995
First published in paperback 1995

A catalogue record for this book is available from the British Library

Library of Congress Cataloging in Publication Data available
ISBN 0 19 262637 X (Hbk)
ISBN 0 19 262670 1 (Pbk)

Typeset by
Interactive Sciences, Gloucester
Printed in Great Britain by
Biddles Ltd, Guildford and King's Lynn

Preface to the Second Edition

This second edition of *Health measurement scales: a practical guide to their development and use* was initiated in recognition of some significant developments in the field of measurement since the first printing in 1989. This in itself is remarkable: psychological measurement is as mature as any of the social sciences, and much of the pioneering work in the field dates to the beginning of the century. That the span of only five years could witness significant changes speaks for the dynamism of the field.

In particular, when we wrote the first edition, generalizability theory, although developed by Cronbach in 1972, was largely a technical curiosity in health measurement. Since then, prompted in part by research efforts surrounding the widespread implementation of the Objective Structured Clinical Examination in North America, generalizablity theory has become an accepted and conventional approach to the investigation of test reliability. As a consequence, whereas the first edition deliberately treated the topic in a cursory manner, in order to merely familiarize the reader with the general concept, the chapter in the present edition (Chapter 9) is much more extensive. Accompanying these changes, we have completely revised Chapter 8 — Reliability — in order to cover new topics and to present these difficult concepts in a more coherent manner.

Measuring change has been a continuing source of debate amongst researchers in measurement for many decades. However, the past decade or so has witnessed a new and elegant approach to the problem, based on individual growth curves, which was initially identified by Rogosa (1981) and has since been refined by a number of investigators. These new techniques are described in Chapter 11.

Ethics in research is not a new topic, but the past decade has witnessed growing concern about the issue, and a number of governmental and non-governmental agencies have issued specific guidelines. Because researchers in measurement must be aware of these issues, a new chapter, Chapter 13, is devoted to a discussion of ethical problems which may be encountered in developing measurement tools.

In addition to these major changes, there have been many minor ones; too many, in fact, for us to list more than a sampling. New sections have been added on Goal Attainment Scaling (GAS) and multidimensional scaling. As is the case with generalizability theory, these are not new techniques, but ones which have seen something of a resurgence in the past few years. On the other hand, the difficulties encountered when two scores (such as the frequency and importance of symptoms) are multiplied together to form a multiplicative composite have only recently been examined in depth, and these are discussed in Chapter 7. We have also expanded the appendix pointing out where to find existing scales to include a wider range of topics and recent additions, and have tried to bring empirical findings on scale development and use up to date.

We have been very gratified by the positive comments we have received about the first edition of this book, and hope that the current edition makes it even more useful to those who want to develop their own scales, or just to learn more about how others have (or should have) gone about this task.

December 1994   D.L.S.
                                                                     G.R.N.

Contents

Appendices

1

Introduction

The act of measurement is an essential component of scientific research, whether in the natural, social, or health sciences.

Until recently, however, discussion regarding issues of measurement was noticeably absent in the deliberations of clinical researchers. Certainly, measurement played as essential a role in research in the health sciences as in other scientific disciplines. However, measurement in the laboratory disciplines presented no inherent difficulty. Like other natural sciences, measurement was a fundamental part of the discipline, and was approached through the development of appropriate instrumentation. Subjective judgement played a minor role in the measurement process; any issue of reproducibility or validity was therefore amenable to a technological solution. It should be mentioned, however, that expensive equipment does not, of itself, eliminate measurement error.

Conversely, clinical researchers were acutely aware of the fallibility of human judgement as evidenced by the errors involved in such processes as radiological diagnosis (Garland 1959; Yerushalmy 1955). Fortunately the research problems approached by many clinical researchers—cardiologists, epidemiologists, and the like—frequently did not depend on subjective assessment. Trials of therapeutic regimens focused on the prolongation of life and the prevention or management of such life-threatening conditions as heart disease, stroke, or cancer. In these circumstances, measurement is reasonably straightforward. 'Objective' criteria, based on laboratory or tissue diagnosis where possible, can be used to decide whether a patient has the disease, and warrants inclusion in the study. The investigator then waits an appropriate period of time and counts those who did or did not survive—and the criteria for death are reasonably well established, even though the exact cause of death may be a little more difficult.

In the past decade or so, the situation in clinical research has become more complex. The effects of new drugs or surgical procedures on *quantity* of life is likely to be marginal indeed. Conversely, there is increased awareness of the impact of health and health care on the *quality* of human life. Therapeutic efforts in many disciplines of medicine—psychiatry, respirology, rheumatology, oncology—other health professions—nursing, physiotherapy, occupational therapy—are directed equally if not primarily to the improvement of quality, not quantity of life. If the efforts of these disciplines are to be placed on a sound scientific basis, methods must be devised to measure what was previously thought to be unmeasurable, and assess in a reproducible and valid fashion those subjective states which cannot be converted into the position of a needle on a dial.

The challenge is not as formidable as it may seem. Psychologists and educators have been grappling with the issue for many years, dating back to the European attempts at the turn of the century to assess individual differences in intelligence (Galton, cited in Allen and Yen 1979; Stern 1979). Since that time, and particularly since the 1930s, much has been accomplished, so that a sound methodology for the development and application of tools to assess subjective states now exists. Unfortunately, much of this literature is virtually unknown to most clinical researchers. Health Science libraries do not routinely catalog *Psychometrica* or *The British Journal of Statistical Psychology*. Nor should they—the language would be incomprehensible to most readers, and the problems of seemingly little relevance.

Similarly, the textbooks in the subject are directed at educational or psychological audiences. The former is concerned with measures of achievement applicable to classroom situations, and the latter is focused primarily on personality or aptitude measures, again with no apparent direct relevance. In general, textbooks in these disciplines are directed to the development of achievement, intelligence or personality tests.

By contrast, researchers in health sciences are frequently faced with the desire to measure something which has not been approached previously—arthritic pain, return to function of post-MI patients, speech difficulties of aphasic stroke patients, or clinical competence of junior medical students. The difficulties and questions raised in developing such instruments range from the straightforward (e.g. 'How many boxes do I put on the response?') to the complex (e.g. 'How do I establish whether the thing is measuring what I hope it is?'). Nevertheless, to a large degree, the answers are known, although frequently difficult to access.

The intent of this book is to introduce researchers in health sciences to these concepts of measurement. It is not an introductory textbook, in that we do not confine ourselves to a discussion of introductory principles and methods; rather, we attempt to make the book as current and comprehensive as possible. The book does not delve as heavily into mathematics as many books in the field; such side trips may provide some intellectual rewards for those so inclined, but frequently at the expense of losing the majority of readers. Similarly, we emphasize applications, rather than theory, so that some theoretical subjects (like Thurstone's Law of Comparative Judgement) which are of historical interest but little practical importance, are omitted. Nevertheless, we spend considerable time in explanation of the concepts underlying current approaches to measurement. One other departure from current books is that our focus is on those attributes of interest to researchers in health sciences—subjective states, attitudes, response to illess, etc. rather than the topics such as personality or achievement familiar to readers in education and psychology. As a result, our examples are drawn from the literature in health sciences.

Finally, some understanding of certain selected topics in statistics is necessary to learn many essential concepts of measurement. In particular, the *correlation coefficient* is used in many empirical studies of measurement instruments. Discussion of reliability is based on the methods of *repeated measures analysis of variance*. Item analysis and certain approaches to test validity use the methods of *factor analysis*. It is not by any means necessary to have detailed knowledge of these methods to understand the concepts of measurement discussed in this book. Still, it would be useful to have some conceptual understanding of these techniques. If the reader requires some review of statistical topics, we have suggested a few appropriate resources in Appendix A.

The book is organized in a sort of chronological sequence; that is, we are attempting to cover topics in the order they might be confronted by someone faced with the problem of developing a new instrument. Chapter 2 provides an overview of the criteria which should be used to assess any measurement instrument; by reviewing this section, the reader should be able to peruse the literature to see if any available instrument is suitable. In the remaining chapters, we assume an unsuccessful search, and provide detailed information regarding the steps involved in developing a new scale. Finally, the appendix provides additional resources for locating further information about issues in measurement, including an annotated bibliography of references for existing scales (Appendix B).

References

Galton, F. (1979). Cited in M. J. Allen and W. M. Yen, *Introduction to Measurement Theory*. Brooks Cole, Monterey.

Garland, L. H. (1959). Studies on the accuracy of diagnostic procedures. *American Journal of Roentgenology*, **82**, 25–38.

Stern, W. (1979). Cited in M. J. Allen and W. M. Yen, *Introduction to Measurement Theory*. Brooks Cole, Monterey.

Yerushalmy, J. (1955). Reliability of chest radiography in diagnosis of pulmonary lesions. *American Journal of Surgery*, **89**, 231–40.

2

Basic concepts

One feature of the health sciences literature devoted to measuring subjective states is the daunting array of available scales. Whether one wishes to measure depression, pain, or patient satisfaction, it seems that every article published in the field has used a different approach to the measurement problem. This proliferation impedes research, since there are significant problems in generalizing from one set of findings to another.

Paradoxically, if you proceed a little further in the search for existing instruments to assess a particular concept, you may conclude that none of the existing scales is quite right, so it is appropriate to embark on the development of one more scale to add to the confusion in the literature. Most researchers tend to magnify the deficiencies of existing measures and underestimate the effort required to develop an adequate new measure. Of course, scales do not exist for all applications; if this were so, there would be little justification for writing this book. Nevertheless, perhaps the most common error committed by clinical researchers is to dismiss existing scales too lightly, and embark on the development of a new instrument with an unjustifiably optimistic and naive expectation that they can do better. As will become evident, the development of scales to assess subjective attributes is not easy and requires considerable investment of both mental and fiscal resources. Therefore, a useful first step is to be aware of any existing scales which might suit the purpose. The next step is to understand and apply criteria for judging the usefulness of a particular scale. In subsequent chapters, these will be described in much greater detail for use in developing a scale; however, the next few pages will serve as an introduction to the topic and a guideline for a critical literature review.

The discussion which follows is necessarily brief. A much more comprehensive set of standards, which is widely used for the assessment of standardized tests used in psychology and education, is the manual called *Standards for educational and psychological tests*, published by the American Psychological Association (1974).

Searching the literature

An initial search of the literature to locate scales for measurement of particular variables might begin with the standard bibliographic sources, particularly Medline. However, depending on the application, one might wish to consider biblio-graphic reference systems in other disciplines, particularly *Psychological Abstracts* for psychological scales and ERIC for instruments designed for edu-cational purposes.

In addition to these standard sources, there are a number of compendia of measuring scales. These are described in Appendix B. We might particularly highlight the volume entitled *Measuring health: A guide to rating scales and questionnaires* (McDowell and Newell 1987) which is a critical review of scales designed to measure a number of characteristics of interest to researchers in the health sciences, such as pain, illness behaviour, and social support.

Critical review

Having located one or more scales of potential interest, it remains to choose whether to use one of these existing scales or to proceed to development of a new instrument. In part this decision can be guided by a judgement of the appro-priateness of the items on the scale, but this should always be supplemented by a critical review of the evidence in support of the instrument. The particular dimensions of this review are described below:

Face and content validity

The terms *face validity* and *content validity* are technical descriptions of the jud-gement that a scale looks reasonable. Face validity simply indicates whether, on the face of it, the instrument appears to be assessing the desired qualities. The criterion represents a subjective judgement based on a review of the measure itself by one or more experts, and rarely are any empirical approaches used. Content validity is a closely related concept, consisting of a judgement whether the instrument samples all the relevant or important content or domains. These two forms of validity consist of a judgement by experts whether the scale appears appropriate for the intended purpose. Guilford (1954) calls this approach to vali-dation 'validity by assumption', meaning the instrument measures such-and-such because an expert says it does. However, an explicit statement regarding face and content validity, based on some form of review by an expert panel or alternative methods described later, should be a minimum prerequisite for acceptance of a measure.

Having said this, there are situations where face and content validity may not be desirable, and may be consciously avoided. For example, in assessing behav-iour such as child abuse or excessive alcohol consumption, questions like 'Have you ever hit your child with a blunt object?' or 'Do you frequently drink to excess?' may have face validity, but are unlikely to elicit an honest response. Questions designed to assess sensitive areas are likely to be less obviously related to the underlying attitude or behaviour, and may appear to have poor face validity. It is rare for scales not to satisfy minimal standards of face and content validity, unless there has been a deliberate attempt from the outset to avoid straightforward questions.

Nevertheless, all too frequently, researchers dismiss existing measures on the basis of their own judgements of face validity—they did not like some of the questions, or the scale was too long, or the responses were not in a preferred format. As we have indicated, this judgement should comprise only one of several used in arriving at an overall judgement of usefulness, and should be balanced against the time and cost of developing a replacement.

Reliability

The concept of *reliability* is, on the surface, deceptively simple. Before one can obtain evidence that an instrument is measuring what is intended, it is first necessary to gather evidence that the scale is measuring *something* in reproducible fashion. That is, a first step in providing evidence of the value of an instrument is to demonstrate that measurements of individuals on different occasions, or by different observers, or by similar or parallel tests, produce the same or similar results.

That is the basic idea behind the concept—an index of the extent to which measurements of individuals obtained under different circumstances yield similar results. However, the concept is refined a bit further in measurement theory. If we were considering the reliability of, for example, a set of bathroom scales, it might be sufficient to indicate that the scales are accurate to ± 1 kg. From this information, we can easily judge whether the scales will be adequate to distinguish among adult males (probably yes) or to assess weight gain of premature infants (probably no), since we have prior knowledge of the average weight and variation in weight of adults and premature infants.

Such information is rarely available in the development of subjective scales. Each scale produces a different measurement from every other. Therefore, to indicate that a particular scale is accurate to ± 3.4 units provides no indication of its value in measuring individuals unless we have some idea about the likely range of scores on the scale. To circumvent this problem, reliability is usually quoted as a ratio of the variability between individuals to the total variability in the scores; in other words, the reliability is a measure of the proportion of the variability in scores which was due to true differences between individuals. Thus, the reliability is expressed as a number between 0 and 1, with 0 indicating no reliability, and 1 indicating perfect reliability.

An important issue in examining the reliability of an instrument is the manner in which the data were obtained which provided the basis for the calculation of a reliability coefficient. First of all, since the reliability involves the ratio of variability between subjects to total variability, one way to ensure that a test will look good is to conduct the study on an extremely heterogeneous sample, for example to measure knowledge of clinical medicine using samples of first year, third year, and fifth year students. Examine the sampling procedures carefully, and assure yourself that the sample used in the reliability study is approximately the same as the sample you wish to study.

Secondly, there are any number of ways in which reliability measures can be obtained, and the magnitude of the reliability coefficient will be a direct reflection of the particular approach used. Some broad definitions are described below:

1. *Internal consistency*. Measures of internal consistency are based on a single administration of the measure. If the measure has a relatively large number of items addressing the same underlying dimension; for example, 'Are you able to dress yourself?', 'Are you able to shop for groceries?', 'Can you do the sewing?' as measures of physical function, then it is reasonable to expect that scores on each item would be correlated with scores on all other items. This is the idea behind measures of internal consistency—essentially, they represent the average of the correlations among all the items in the measure. There are a number of ways to calculate these correlations, called *Cronbach's alpha*, *Kuder–Richardson*, or *split halves*, but all yield similar results. Since the method involves only a single administration of the test, such coefficients are easy to obtain. However, they do not take into account any variation from day to day or from observer to observer, and thus lead to an optimistic interpretation of the true reliability of the test.

2. *Stability*. There are a variety of ways of examining the reproduceability of a measure administered on different occasions. For example, one might ask about the degree of agreement between different observers (*inter-observer reliability*); the agreement between observations made by the same rater on two different occasions (*intra-observer reliability*); observations on the patient on two occasions separated by some interval of time (*test–retest reliability*), and so forth. As a minimum, any decision regarding the value of a measure should be based on some information regarding stability of the instrument. Internal consistency, in its many guises, is not a sufficient basis upon which to make a reasoned judgement.

3. *Standards of acceptable reliability*. One difficulty with the reliability coefficient is that it is simply a number between 0 and 1, and does not lend itself to commonsense interpretations. Various authors have made different recommendations regarding the minimum accepted level of reliability. Certainly, internal consistency should exceed 0.8, and it might be reasonable to demand stability measures greater than 0.5. Depending on the use of the test, and the cost of misinterpretation, higher values might be required.

Finally, although there is a natural concern that many instruments in the literature are too long to be practical, the reason for the length should be borne in mind. If we assume that every response has some associated error of measurement, then by averaging or summing responses over a series of questions, we can reduce this error. For example, if the original test has a reliability of 0.5, doubling the test will increase the reliability to 0.67, and quadrupling it will result in a reliability of 0.8. As a result, we must recognize that there is a very good reason for long tests; brevity is not necessarily a desirable attribute of a test, and is achieved at some cost.

Empirical forms of validity

Reliability simply assesses that a test is measuring something in a reproducible fashion; it says nothing about *what* is being measured. To determine that the test is measuring what was intended requires some evidence of 'validity'. To demonstrate validity requires more than peer judgements; empirical evidence must be produced to show that the tool is measuring what is intended. How is this achieved?

Although there are many approaches to assessing validity, and myriad terms used to describe these approaches, eventually the situation reduces to two circumstances:

1. *Other scales of the same or similar attributes are available.* In the situation where measures already exist, then an obvious approach is to administer the experimental instrument and one of the existing instruments to a sample of people and see whether there is a strong correlation between the two. As an example, there are many scales to measure depression. In developing a new scale, it is straightforward to administer the new and old instruments to the same sample. This approach is described by several terms in the literature including *convergent validity*, *criterion validity*, and *concurrent validity*. The distinction among the terms will be made clear in Chapter 10.

Although this method is straightforward it has two severe limitations. First, if other measures of the same property already exist, then it is difficult to justify developing yet another unless it is cheaper or simpler. Of course, many researchers believe that the new instrument that they are developing is better than the old, which provides an interesting bit of circular logic. If the new method is better than the old, why compare it to the old method? And if the relationship between the new method and the old is less than perfect, which one is at fault?

In fact, the nature of the measurement challenges we are discussing in this book usually precludes the existence of any conventional 'gold standard'. Although there are often measures which have, through history or longevity, acquired criterion status, a close review usually suggests that they have less than ideal reliability and validity. Any measurement we are likely to make will have some associated error; as a result we should expect that correlations among measures of the same attribute should fall in the midrange of 0.4–0.8. Any lower correlation suggests that either the reliability of one or the other measure is likely unacceptably low, or that they are measuring different phenomena.

2. *No other measure exists.* This situation is the more likely, since it is usually the justification for developing a scale in the first instance. At first glance, though, we seem to be confronting an impossible situation. After all, if no measure

exists, how can one possibly acquire data to show that the new measure is indeed measuring what is intended?

The solution lies in a broad set of approaches labelled *construct validity*. We begin by linking the attribute we are measuring to some other attribute by a hypothesis or construct. Usually this hypothesis will explore the difference between two or more populations who would be expected to have differing amounts of the property assessed by our instrument. We then test this hypothetical construct by applying our instrument to the appropriate samples. If the expected relationship is found, then the hypothesis and the measure are sound; conversely, if no relationship is found, the fault may lie with either the measure or the hypothesis.

Let us clarify this with an example. Suppose that the year is 1920, and a biochemical test of blood sugar has just been devised. Enough is known to hypothesize that diabetics have higher blood sugar values than normal subjects; but no other test of blood sugar exists. Here are some likely hypotheses which could be tested empirically:

- Individuals diagnosed as diabetic on clinical criteria will have higher blood sugar on the new test than comparable controls.

- Dogs whose pancreases are removed will show increasing levels of blood sugar in the days from surgery until death.

- Individuals who have sweet-tasting urine will have higher blood sugar than those who do not.

- Diabetics injected with insulin extract will show a decrease in blood sugar levels following the injection.

These hypotheses certainly do not exhaust the number of possibilities, but each can be put to an experimental test. Further, it is evident that we should not demand a perfect relationship between blood sugar and the other variable, or even that each and all relationships are significant. But the weight of the evidence should be in favour of a positive relationship.

Similar constructs can be developed for almost any instrument, and in the absence of a concurrent test, some evidence of construct validity should be available. However, the approach is non-specific, and is unlikely to result in very strong relationships. Therefore, the burden of evidence in testing construct validity arises not from a single powerful experiment, but from a series of converging experiments.

The two traditions of assessment

Not surprisingly, medicine on the one hand and psychology and education on the other have developed different ways of evaluating people; ways that have influenced how and why assessment tools are constructed in the first place, and the manner in which they are interpreted. This has led each camp to ignore the potential contribution of the other: the physicians contending that the psycho-metricians do not appreciate how the results must be used to abet clinical decision making, and the psychologists and educators accusing the physicians of ignoring many of the basic principles of test construction, such as reliability and validity. It has only been within the last decade that some rapprochement has been reached; a mutual recognition that we feel is resulting in clinical instru-ments which are both psychometrically sound as well as clinically useful. In this section, we will explore two of these different starting points—categorical versus dimensional conceptualization and the reduction of measurement error—and see how they are being merged.

Categorical versus dimensional conceptualization

Medicine traditionally has thought in terms of diagnoses and treatments. In the most simplistic terms, a patient either has a disorder or does not, and is either prescribed some form of treatment or is not. Thus, diastolic blood pressure (DBP), which is measured on a continuum of millimetres of mercury, is often broken down into just two categories: normotensive (under 90 mm in North America), in which case nothing needs to be done; and hypertensive (90 mm and above), which calls for some form of intervention.

Test constructors who come from the realm of psychology and education, though, look to the writings of S. Smith Stevens (1951) as received wisdom. He introduced the concept of 'levels of measurement', which categorizes variables as *nominal*, *ordinal*, *interval*, or *ratio*—a concept we will return to in greater depth in Chapter 4. The basic idea is that the more finely we can measure some-thing, the better; rating an attribute on a scale in which each point is equally spaced from its neighbours is vastly superior to dividing the attribute into rougher categories with fewer divisions. Thus, psychometricians tend to think of attributes as continua, with people falling along the dimension in terms of how much of the attribute they have.

The implications of these two different ways of thinking have been summar-ized by Devins (1993), and are presented in modified form in Table 2.1. In the categorical mode, the diagnosis of, for example, major depression in the *Diag-nostic and statistical manual* (DMS-IIIR; American Psychiatric Association 1987) requires that the person exhibit at least five of nine symptoms (one of which, depressed mood or loss of interest/pleasure, must be among the five) and that none of four exclusion criteria be present. In turn, each of the symptoms, such as weight change or sleep disturbance, has its own minimum criterion for being judged to be demonstrated (the threshold value). A continuous measure of depression, such as the Center for Epidemiological Studies – Depression scale (CES-D; Radloff 1977), uses a completely different approach. There are 20 items, each scored 1 through 4, and a total score over 16 is indicative of depression. No specific item must be endorsed, and there are numerous ways that a score of 16 can be achieved—a person can have four items rated 4, or 16

Table 2.1 *Categorical and dimensional conceptualization*

	Categorical model	Dimensional model
1.	Diagnosis requires that multiple criteria, each with its threshold value, be satisfied.	Occurrence of some features at high intensities can compensate for non-occurrence of others.
2.	Phenomenon differs qualitatively and quantitatively at different severities.	Phenomenon differs only quantitatively, at different severities.
3.	Differences between cases and non-cases are implicit in the definition.	Differences between cases and non-cases are less clearly delineated.
4.	Severity is lowest in instances that minimally satisfy diagnostic criteria.	Severity is lowest among non-disturbed individuals.
5.	One diagnosis often precludes others.	A person can have varying amounts of different disorders.

items rated 1, or any combination in between. Thus, for diagnostic purposes, having many mild symptoms is equivalent to having a few severe ones.

Second, DSM-IIIR differentiates among various types of depressions according to their severity and course. A bipolar depression is qualitatively and quantitatively different from a dysthymic disorder; different sets of criteria must be met to reflect that the former is not only more severe than the latter, but that it is cyclical in its time course, whereas dysthymia is not. On the other hand, the CES-D quantifies the depressive symptomatology, but does not differentiate among the various types. Consequently, it would reflect that one person's symptoms may be more extensive than another's, irrespective of category.

One implication of this difference is that there is a clear distinction between cases and non-cases with the categorical approach, but not with the dimensional. In the former, one either meets the criteria and is a case, or else the criteria are not satisfied, and one is not a case. With the latter, 'caseness' is a matter of degree, and there is no clear dividing line. The use of a cut point on the CES-D is simply a strategy so that it can be used as a diagnostic tool. The value of 16 was chosen only because, based on empirical findings, using this score maximized agreement between the CES-D and clinical diagnosis; the number is not based on any theoretical argument. Furthermore, there would be less difference seen between two people, one of whom has a score of 15 and the other 17, than between two other people with scores of 30 and 40, although one is a 'case' and the other not in the first instance, and both would be 'cases' in the second.

Another implication is that, since people who do not meet the criteria are said to be free of the disorder with the categorical approach, differences in severity are seen only among those who are diagnosed (point 4 in Table 2.1). Quantification of severity is implicit, with the assumption that those who meet more of the criteria have a more severe depression than people who satisfy only the minimum number. With the dimensional approach, even 'normal' people may have measurable levels of depressive symptomatology; a non-depressed person whose sleep is restless would score higher on the CES-D than a non-depressed person without sleep difficulties.

Last, using the categorical approach, it is difficult (at least within psychiatry) for a person to have more than one disorder. A diagnosis of major depression, for example, cannot be made if the patient has a psychotic condition, or shows evidence of delusions or hallucinations. The dimensional approach does permit this; some traits may be present, albeit in a mild form, even when others coexist.

The limitations of adhering strictly to one or the other of these ways of thinking are becoming more evident. The categorical mode of thinking is starting to change, in part due to the expansion of the armamentarium of treatment options. Returning to the example of hypertension, now patients can be started on salt-restricted diets, followed by diuretics at higher levels of the DBP, and finally placed on vasodilators. Consequently, it makes more sense to measure blood pressure on a continuum, and to titrate the type and amount of treatment to smaller differences, than to simply dichotomize the reading. On the other hand, there are different treatment implications, depending on whether one has a bipolar or a non-cyclical form of depression. Simply measuring the severity of symptomatology does not allow for this. One resolution, which will be discussed in Chapter 4, called multidimensional scaling, is an attempt to bridge these two traditions. It permits a variety of attributes to be measured dimensionally, in such a way that the results can be used to both categorize and determine the extent to which these categories are present.

The reduction of measurement error

Whenever definitive laboratory tests do not exist, physicians rely primarily on the clinical interview to provide differential diagnoses. The clinician is the person who both elicits the information and interprets its significance as a sign or symptom (Dohrenwend and Dohrenwend 1982). Measurement error is reduced through training, interviewing skills, and especially clinical experience. Thus, older physicians are often regarded as 'gold standards', since they presumably have more experience and therefore would make fewer errors. (In a different context, though, Caputo (1980) wrote, 'They haven't got seventeen years' experience, just one year's experience repeated seventeen times' (p. 370).)

In contrast, the psychometric tradition relies on self-reports of patients to usually close-ended questions. It is assumed that the response to any one question is subject to error: the person may misinterpret the item, respond in a biased manner, or make a mistake in transcribing his or her reply to the answer sheet. The effect of these errors is minimized in a variety of ways. First, each item is screened to determine if it meets certain criteria. Second, the focus is on the consistency of the answers across many items, and for the most part, disregarding the responses to the individual questions. Last, the scale as a whole is checked to see if it meets another set of criteria.

The 'medical' approach is often criticized as placing unwarranted faith in the clinical skills of the interviewer. Indeed, as was mentioned briefly in Chapter 1, the reliability (and hence the validity) of the clinical interview leaves much to be desired. Conversely, psychometrically sound tests may provide reliable and valid data, but do not yield the rich clinical information and the ways in which patients differ from one another which come from talking to them in a conversational manner. These two 'solitudes' are starting to merge, especially in psychiatry, as is seen in some of the more recent structured interviews, such as the Diagnostic Interview Schedule (DIS; Robins *et al*. 1981). The DIS is derived from the clinical examination used to diagnose psychiatric patients, but is constructed in such a way that it can be administered by trained lay people, not just psychiatrists. It also relies on the necessity of answering a number of questions before an attribute is judged to be present. Thus, elements of both traditions guided its construction, although purists from both camps will be dissatisfied with the compromises.

Summary

The criteria we have described are intended as a guideline for reviewing the literature, and as an introduction to the remainder of this book. We must emphasize that the research enterprise involved in development of a new method of measurement requires time and patience. Effort expended to locate an existing measure is justified, because of the savings if one can be located and the additional insights provided in the development of a new instrument if none prove satisfactory.

References

American Psychiatric Association (1987). *Diagnostic and statistical manual of mental disorders* (3rd edn., revised). American Psychiatric Association, Washington DC.

American Psychological Association (1985). *Standards for educational and psychological testing*. American Psychological Association, Washington.

Caputo, P. (1980). *Horn of Africa*. Holt, Rinehart and Winston, New York.

Devins, G. (1993). *Psychiatric rating scales*. Paper presented at the Clarke Institute of Psychiatry, Toronto, Ontario.

Dohrenwend, B. P. and Dohrenwend, B. S. (1982). Perspectives on the past and future of psychiatric epidemiology. *American Journal of Public Health*, **72**, 1271–9.

Guilford, J. P. (1954). *Psychometric methods*. McGraw-Hill, New York.

McDowell, I. and Newell, C. (1987). *Measuring Health*. Oxford University Press, Oxford.

Radloff, L. S. (1977). The CES-D scale: A self-report depression scale for research in the general population. *Applied Psychological Measurement*, **1**, 385–401.

Robins, L. N., Helzer, J. E., Crougham, R., and Ratcliff, K. S. (1981). National Institute of Mental Health Diagnostic Interview Schedule: Its history, characteristics, and validity. *Archives of General Psychiatry*, **38**, 381–9.

Stevens, S. S. (1951). Mathematics, measurement, and psychophysics. In *Handbook of experimental psychology* (ed. S. S. Stevens) pp. 1–49. Wiley, New York.

3

Devising the items

The first step in writing a scale or questionnaire is, naturally, devising the items themselves. This is far from a trivial task, since no amount of statistical manipulation after the fact can compensate for poorly chosen questions; those that are badly worded, ambiguous, irrelevant, or—even worse—not present. In this chapter we explore various sources of items, and the strengths and weaknesses of each of them.

The first step is to look at what others have done in the past. Instruments rarely spring full grown from the brows of their developers. Rather, they are usually based on what other people have deemed to be relevant, important, or discriminating. Wechsler (1958), for example, quite openly discussed the patrimony of the subtests which were later incorporated into his various IQ tests. Of the 11 subtests which comprise the adult version, at least nine were derived from other widely used indices. Moreover, the specific items which make up the individual subtests are themselves based on older tests. Both the items and the subtests were modified and new ones added to meet his requirements, but in many cases the changes were relatively minor. Similarly, the *Manifest Anxiety Scale* (Taylor 1953) is based in large measure on one scale from the *Minnesota Multiphasic Personality Inventory* (MMPI; Hathaway and McKinley 1951).

The long, and sometimes tortuous, path by which items from one test end up in others is beautifully described by Goldberg (1971). He wrote that:

Items devised around the turn of the century may have worked their way via Woodworth's Personal Data Sheet, to Thurstone and Thurstone's Personality Schedule, hence to Bernreuter's Personality Inventory, and later to the Minnesota Multiphasic Personality Inventory, where they were borrowed for the California Personality Inventory and then injected into the Omnibus Personality Inventory—only to serve as a source of items for the new Academic Behavior Inventory (p. 335)

which Angleitner *et al.* (1986) expanded to, 'and, we may add, only to be translated and included in some new German personality inventories' (p. 66).

There are a number of reasons that items are repeated from previous inventories. First, it saves work and the necessity of constructing new ones. Second, the items have usually gone through repeated processes of testing, so that they have proven themselves to be useful and psychometrically sound. Third, there are only a limited number of ways to ask about a specific problem. If we were trying to tap depressed mood, for instance, it is difficult to ask about sleep loss in a way that hasn't been used previously.

Hoary as this tradition may be, there are (at least) two problems in adopting it uncritically. First, it may result in items which use outdated terminology. For example, the original version of the MMPI (in use until 1987) contained such quaint terms such as 'deportment', 'cutting up', and 'drop the handkerchief'. Endorsement of these items most likely told more about the person's age than about any aspect of his or her personality. Perhaps more importantly, the motivation for developing a new tool is the investigator's belief that the previous scales are inadequate for one reason or another, or do not completely cover the domain under study. At this point, new items can come from five different sources: the patients or subjects themselves, clinical observation, theory, research, and expert opinion, although naturally the lines between these categories are not firm.

The source of items

A point often overlooked in scale development is the fact that patients and potential research subjects are an excellent source of items. Whereas clinicians may be the best observers of the outward manifestations of a trait or disorder, only those who have it can report on the more subjective elements. Over the years, a variety of techniques have been developed which can elicit these viewpoints in a rigorous and systematic manner; these procedures are used primarily by 'qualitative' researchers, and are only now finding their way into more 'quantitative' types of studies. Here, we can touch only briefly on two of the more relevant techniques; greater detail is provided in texts such as Taylor and Bogden (1984) and Willms and Johnson (1993).

Focus groups

Willms and Johnson (1993) describe a focus group as:

. . . a discussion in which a small group of informants (six to twelve people), guided by a facilitator, talk freely and spontaneously about themes considered important to the investigation. The participants are selected from a target group whose opinions and ideas are of interest to the researcher. Sessions are usually tape recorded and an observer (recorder) also takes notes on the discussion (p. 61).

In the area of scale development, the participants would be patients who have the disorder, or subjects representative of those whose opinions would be elicited by the instrument. At first, their task would not be to generate the specific items, but rather to suggest general themes which the research team can use to phrase the items themselves. Usually, no more than two or three groups would be needed. Once the items have been written, focus groups can again be used to discuss whether these items are relevant, clear, unambiguous, written in terms that are understood by potential respondents, and if all the main themes have been covered. These groups are much more focused than during the theme generation stage, since there is a strong externally generated agenda; discussing the items themselves.

Key informant interviews

As the name implies, these are indepth interviews with a small number of people, chosen because of their unique knowledge. These can be patients who have or have had the disorder, for example, and who can articulate what they felt; or clinicians who have extensive experience with the patients and can explain it from their perspective. The interviews can range from informal or unstructured ones, which are almost indistinguishable from spontaneous conversations, to highly structured ones, where the interviewer has a preplanned set of carefully worded questions. Generally, the less that is known about the area under study, the less structured the interview. There is no set number of people who should be interviewed. The criterion often used in this type of research is 'sampling to redundancy'; that is, interviewing people until no new themes emerge.

Clinical observation is perhaps one of the most fruitful sources of items. Indeed, it can be argued that observation, whether of patients or students, precedes theory, research, or expert opinion. Scales are simply a way of gathering these clinical observations in a systematic fashion, so that all observers are ensured of looking for the same thing, or all subjects of responding to the same items. As an example, Kruis *et al.* (1984) devised a scale to try to differentiate between irritable bowel syndrome (IBS) and organic bowel disease. The first part of their questionnaire consists of a number of items asked by the clinician of the patient—presence of abdominal pain and flatulence, alteration in bowel habits, duration of symptoms, type and intensity of pain, abnormality of the stools, and so forth. The choice of these items was predicated on the clinical experience of the authors, and their impressions of how IBS patients' symptomatology and presentation differ from other patients'. Similarly, the *Menstrual Distress Questionnaire* (Moos 1984) consists of 47 symptoms, such as muscle stiffness, skin blemishes, fatigue, and feeling sad or blue, which have been reported clinically to be associated with premenstrual syndrome (PMS).

This is not to say that these groups of researchers are necessarily correct, in that the items they selected *are* different between patients with organic or functional bowel disease, or between women who do and do not have PMS. In fact, perhaps the major drawback of relying solely on clinical observation to guide the selection of items is the real possibility that the clinicians may be wrong. The original rationale for electroconvulsive shock therapy, for instance, was based on a quite erroneous 'observation' that the incidence of epilepsy is far lower in the schizophrenic population than with normals. Any scale which tried to capitalize on this association would be doomed to failure. A related problem is that the clinician, because of a limited sample of patients, or narrow perspective imposed by a particular model of the disorder, may not be aware of other factors which may prove to be better descriptors or discriminators.

Clinical observation rarely exists in isolation. Individual laboratory results or physical findings convey far more information if they are components of a more global theory of an illness or behaviour. The term *theory*, in this context, is used very broadly, encompassing not only formal, refutable models of how things relate to one another, but also to vaguely formed hunches of how or why people behave, if only within a relatively narrow domain. A postulate that patients who believe in the efficacy of therapy will be more compliant with their physician's orders, for example, may not rival the theory of relativity in its scope or predictive power, but can be a fruitful source of items in this limited area. A theory or model can thus serve a heuristic purpose, suggesting items or subscales.

At first glance, it may appear as if theory is what we rely on until data are available; once studies have been done, it would be unnecessary to resort to theory and the scale developer can use facts to generate items or guide construction of the scale. Indeed, this was the prevailing attitude among test designers until relatively recently. However, there has been an increasing appreciation of the role that theory can play in scale and questionnaire development. This is seen most clearly when we are trying to assess attitudes, beliefs, or traits. For example, if we wanted to devise a scale which could predict those post-MI patients who would comply with an exercise regimen, our task would be made easier (and perhaps more accurate) if we had some model or theory of compliance. The Health Belief Model (Becker *et al.* 1979), for instance, postulates that compliance is a function of numerous factors, including the patient's perception of the severity of the disorder and his susceptibility to it, and his belief in the effectiveness of the proposed therapy, as well as external cues to comply and barriers which may impede compliance. If this model has any validity, then it would make sense for the scale to include items from each of these areas, some of which may not have occurred to the investigator without the model.

The obverse side is that a model which is wrong can lead us astray, prompting us to devise questions which ultimately have no predictive or explanatory power. While the inadequacy of the theory may emerge later in testing the validity of the scale, much time and effort can be wasted in the interim. For example, Patient Management Problems (PMPs) were based on the supposition that physician competence is directly related to the thoroughness and comprehensiveness of the history and physical examination. The problems, therefore, covered every conceivable question that could be asked of a patient and most laboratory tests that could be ordered. The scoring system similarly reflected this theory; points were gained by being obsessively compulsive, and lost if the right diagnosis were arrived at by the 'wrong' route, one which used short cuts. While psychometrically sound, the PMPs did not correlate with any other measure of clinical competence, primarily for the reason that the model was wrong—expert physicians do not function in the way envisioned by the test developers (Feightner 1985).

Just as naked observations need the clothing of a theory, so a theory must ultimately be tested empirically. *Research findings* can be a fruitful source of items and subscales. For the purposes of scale construction, research can be of two types; a literature review of studies which have been done in the area, or new research carried out specifically for the purpose of developing the scale. In both cases, the scale or questionnaire would be comprised of items which have been shown empirically to be characteristic of a group of people, or which differentiate them from other people.

As an example of a scale based on previous research, the second part of the Kruis *et al.* (1984) scale for IBS is essentially a checklist of laboratory values and clinical history; e.g. erythrocyte sedimentation rate, leucocytosis, and weight loss. These were chosen on the basis of previous research which indicated that IBS and organic patients differed on these variables. This part of the scale, then, is a summary of empirical findings based on research done by others.

In a different domain, Ullman and Giovannoni (1964) developed a scale to measure the 'process—reactive' continuum in schizophrenia. A number of items on the questionnaire relate to marriage and parenthood, because there is considerable evidence that process schizophrenics, especially males, marry at a far lower rate than do reactive schizophrenics. Another item relates to alcohol consumption, since among schizophrenics at least, those who use alcohol tend to have shorter hospital stays than those who do not drink.

When entering into a new area, though, there may not be any research which can serve as the basis for items. Under these circumstances, it may be necessary for the scale developer to conduct some preliminary research, which can then be the source of items. For example, Brumback and Howell (1972) needed an index to evaluate the clinical effectiveness of physicians working in federal hospitals and clinics. Existing scales were inadequate or inappropriate for their purposes, and did not provide the kind of information they needed in a format which was acceptable to the raters. The checklist portion of the scale they ultimately developed was derived by gathering 2500 descriptions of critical incidents from 500 people; classifying these into functional areas; and then using various item analytic techniques (to be discussed in Chapter 6) to arrive at the final set of 37 items. While this study is unusual in its size, it illustrates two points. First, it is sometimes necessary to perform research prior to constructing the scale itself in order to determine key aspects of the domain under investigation. Second, the initial item pool is often much larger than the final set of items. Again, the size of the reduction is quite unusual in this study (only 1.5 per cent of the original items were ultimately retained), but the fact that reduction occurs is not.

The use of *expert opinion* in a given field was illustrated in a similar study by Cowles and Kubany (1959) to evaluate the performance of medical students. Experienced faculty members were interviewed to determine what they felt were the most important characteristics students should have in preparing for general practice, ultimately resulting in eight items. This appears quite similar to the first step taken by Brumback and Howell, which was labelled 'research'; indeed, the line between the two is a very fine one and the distinction somewhat arbitrary.

The important point is that, in both cases, information had to be gathered prior to the construction of the scale.

There are no hard and fast rules governing the use of expert judgements: how many experts to use, how they are found and chosen, or even more important, how differences among them are reconciled. The methods by which the opinions are gathered can run the gamut from having a colleague scribble some comments on a rough draft of the questionnaire to holding a conference of recognized leaders in the field, with explicit rules governing voting. Most approaches usually fall between these two extremes; somewhere in the neighbourhood of three to ten people known to the scale developer as experts are consulted, usually individually. Since the objective is to generate as many potential items as possible for the scale, those suggested by even one person should be considered, at least in the first draft of the instrument.

The advantage of this approach is that if the experts are chosen carefully, they probably represent the most recent thinking in an area. Without much effort, the scale developer has access to the accumulated knowledge and experience of others who have worked in the field. The disadvantages may arise if the panel is skewed in some way, and does not reflect a range of opinions. Then, the final selection of items may represent one particular viewpoint, and there may be glaring gaps in the final product.

It should be borne in mind that these are not mutually exclusive methods of generating items. A scale may consist of items derived from some or all of these sources. Indeed, it would be unusual to find any questionnaire derived from only one of them.

Content validity

Once the items have been generated from these various sources, the scale developer is ideally left with far more items than will ultimately end up on the scale. In Chapter 5 we will discuss various statistical techniques to select the best items from this pool. For the moment, though, we address the converse of this, ensuring that the scale has enough items and adequately covers the domain under investigation. The technical term for this is *content validity*, although some theorists have argued that 'content relevance' and 'content coverage' would be more accurate descriptors (Messick 1980). These concepts arose from achievement testing, where students are assessed to determine if they have learned the material in a specific content area; final examinations are the prime example. With this in mind, each item on the test should relate to one of the course objectives (content relevance). Items which are not related to the content of the course introduce error in the measurement, in that they discriminate among the students on some dimension other than the one purportedly tapped by the test; a dimension that can be totally irrelevant to the test. Conversely, each part of the syllabus should be represented by one or more questions (content coverage). If

Table 3.1 *Checking content validity for a course in cardiology*

Question	Content Area				
	Anatomy	Physiology	Function	...	Pathology
1		×			
2	×				
3			×		
4	×				
5					×
.					
.					
.					
20		×			

not, then students may differ in some important respects, but this would not be reflected in the final score. Table 3.1 shows how these two components of content validity can be checked in a course of, for example, cardiology. Each row reflects a different item on the test, and each column a different content area. Every item is examined in turn, and a mark placed in the appropriate column(s). Although a single number does not emerge at the end, as with other types of validity estimates, the visual display yields much information.

First, each item should fall into at least one content area represented by the columns. If it does not, then either that item is not relevant to the course objectives, or the list of objectives is not comprehensive. Second, each objective should be represented by at least one question; otherwise, it is not being evaluated by the test. Last, the number of questions in each area should reflect its actual importance in the syllabus. The reason for checking this is that it is quite simple to write items in some areas, and far more difficult in others. In cardiology, for example, it is much easier to write multiple-choice items to find out if the students know the normal values of obscure enzymes than to devise questions tapping their ability to deal with the rehabilitation of cardiac patients. Thus, there may be a disproportionately large number of the former items on the test and too few of the latter in relation to what the students should know. The final score, then, would not be an accurate reflection of what the instructor hoped the students would learn.

Depending on how finely one defines the course objectives, it may not be possible to assess each one, as this would make the test too long. Under these conditions, it would be necessary to *randomly sample* the domain of course objectives; that is, select them in such a way that each has an equal opportunity of being chosen. This indeed is closer to what is often done in measuring traits or behaviours, since tapping the full range of them may make the instrument unwieldy.

Although this matrix method was first developed for achievement tests, it can be applied equally well to scales measuring attitudes, behaviours, symptoms, and the like. In these cases, the columns are comprised of aspects of the trait or disorder that the investigator wants the scale to cover, rather than course objectives. Assume, for example, that the test constructor wanted to develop a new measure to determine whether living in a home insulated with urea formaldehyde foam (UFFI) leads to physical problems. The columns in this case would be those areas she felt would be affected by UFFI (and perhaps a few that should *not* be affected, if she wanted to check on a general tendency to endorse symptoms). So, based on previous research, theory, expert opinion and other sources, these may include upper respiratory symptoms, gastrointestinal complaints, skin rash, sleep disturbances, memory problems, eye irritation, and so forth. This would then serve as a check that all domains were covered by at least one question, and that there were no irrelevant items. As can be seen, content validity applies to the scale as a whole, not to the separate items individually.

Let us use a concrete example to illustrate how these various steps are put into practice. As part of a study to examine the effects of stress (McFarlane *et al.* 1980), a scale was needed to measure the amount of social support that the respondents felt they had. Although there were a number of such instruments already in existence, none met the specific needs of this project, or matched closely enough our theoretical model of social support. Thus, the first step, although not clearly articulated as such at the time, was to elucidate our *theory* of social support; what areas we wanted to tap, and which we felt were irrelevant or unnecessary for our purposes. This was augmented by *research* done in the field by other groups, indicating aspects of social support which served as buffers, protecting the person against stress. The next step was to locate *previous instruments*, and cull from them those questions or approaches which met our needs. Finally, we showed a preliminary draft of our scale to a number of highly experienced family therapists, whose *expert opinion* was formed on the basis of their years of *clinical observation*. This last step actually served two related purposes: they performed a *content validity* study, seeing if any important areas were missed by us, and also suggested additional items to fill these gaps. The final draft (McFarlane *et al.* 1981) was then subjected to a variety of reliability and validity checks, as outlined in subsequent chapters.

Generic versus specific scales and the 'fidelity versus bandwidth' issue

Let us say you want to find or develop a test to measure the quality of life (QOL) of a group of rheumatoid arthritis patients. Should you look for (or develop) a QOL instrument which is tailored to the characteristics of these RA patients, or should it be a scale which taps QOL for patients with a variety of disorders, of which RA is only one? Indeed, should we go even further, and tailor the scale to the unique requirements of the individual patients? There are some scales (e.g.

Guyatt *et al.* 1993) which are constructed by asking the patient to list five activities which he or she feels have been most affected by the disorder. Thus, this item on one patient's scale may be quite different from those on anyone else's instrument.

The argument in favour of disease-specific and patient-specific questionnaires is twofold. The first consideration is that if an instrument has to cover a wide range of disorders, many of the questions may be inappropriate or irrelevant for any one specific problem. A generic scale, for example, may include items tapping incontinence, shortness of breath, and problems in attention and concentration. These are areas which may present difficulties for patients with Crohn's disease, asthma, or depression, but rarely for arthritics. Consequently, these non-useful items contribute nothing but noise when the questionnaire is used for one specific disorder. This argument is simply carried to its logical extreme with patient-specific instruments; here, all of the items are, by definition, relevant for the patient, and there should be no items which are not applicable, or should not change with effective therapy.

The second reason for using disease- or patient-specific scales follows directly from the first problem. In order to keep the length of a generic questionnaire manageable, there cannot be very many items in each of the areas tapped. Thus, there will be fewer relevant questions to detect real changes within patients, or differences among them.

On the opposite side of the argument, the cost of the greater degree of specificity is a reduction in generalizability (Aaronson 1988, 1989). That is, generic scales allow comparisons across different disorders, severities of disease, interventions, and perhaps even demographic and cultural groups (Patrick and Deyo 1989), as well as being able to measure the burden of illness of populations suffering from chronic medical and psychiatric conditions as compared with normals (McHorney *et al.* 1994). This is much harder, or even impossible, to do when each study uses a different scale. Especially in light of the recent increase in the use of meta-analysis to synthesize the results of different studies (e.g. Glass *et al.* 1981), this can be a major consideration. Furthermore, since any one generic scale tends to be used more frequently than a given specific instrument, there are usually more data available regarding its reliability and validity.

These problems are even more acute with patient-specific scales. Since no two people have exactly the same scale, it is difficult to establish psychometric properties such as reliability and validity, or to make any comparisons across people, much less across different disorders. Another problem is a bit more subtle. Since all patients choose their most troublesome symptoms, this means that they will all start off with very similar scores, even if they differ among themselves quite considerably in other areas. That is, even if Patient A has problems in six areas, and Patient B in 11, they will be identical on the scale if each can choose only the five most bothersome. Furthermore, since they both will start off at the test's ceiling, they have nowhere to go but down, making any intervention look effective.

Another way of conceptualizing the difference between specific and generic scales is related to what Cronbach (1990) labelled the 'bandwidth versus fidelity' dilemma. The term comes from communication theory (Shannon and Weaver 1949), and refers to the problem faced in designing radios. If we build a receiver that covers all of the AM and FM stations, plus the short-wave bands, and also allows us to monitor police and fire calls, then we have achieved a wide bandwidth. The trade-off, though, is that no one station is heard very well. The opposite extreme is to design a receiver that will pick up only one station. The fidelity of the reception will be superb since all of the components are designed for that one specific part of the spectrum, but the radio will be useless for any other station we may want to hear. Thus, we achieve bandwidth at the cost of fidelity, and vice versa.

The issue is the proper balance between a narrow scale with low bandwidth and (presumably) good fidelity versus a generic scale with greater bandwidth but (again presumably) poorer fidelity. The literature comparing these two types of scales is somewhat limited. However, the general conclusion is that the advantages of disease-specific scales may be more apparent than real; well-designed, reliable, and valid generic questionnaires appear to yield results at least as good as, and often better than, disease-specific ones across a number of illnesses and instruments (e.g. Bombardier *et al.* 1986; Liang *et al.* 1985; Parkerson *et al.* 1993).

Translation

Although it is not directly related to the problem of devising items, translation into another language is a problem that may have to be addressed. In most large studies, especially those located in major metropolitan centres, it is quite probable that English will not be the first language of a significant proportion of respondents. This raises one of two possible alternatives, both of which have associated problems. First, such respondents can be eliminated from the study. However, this raises the possibility that the sample will then not be a representative one, and the results may have limited generalizability. The second alternative is to translate the scales and questionnaires into the languages most commonly used within the catchment area encompassed by the study.

The translation process itself is a complex one, and may introduce subtle forms of distortions into the scale. The first step consists of translating the individual items or questions into the other language. This is best done by someone who is not only fluent in both English and the target tongue, but who is also knowledgeable about the content area, and is aware of the intent of each item and of the scale as a whole. The reason is that the literal translation of phrases may convey very different meanings in the two languages; feelings, disorders, and even symptoms may not be expressed in the same manner in other cultures. For example, we generally associate the colour blue with sadness, and black with depression. In China, though, white is the colour of mourning, a shade we use to connote purity. Consequently, a literal translation of the phrase, 'I feel blue,' or 'The future looks black to me' may generate a response, but the meaning of the answer would be problematic. Similarly, Anglo-Saxons often associate mild physical discomfort with stomach problems, whereas the French would be more prone to attribute it to their liver, and Germans to their circulation.

A more subtle problem is that the meaning of the construct that the scale is to tap may differ from culture to culture. For example, before translating a scale of child abuse into Spanish, one of our students (Aracena *et al.* 1994) decided to conduct some focus groups to determine if the meaning of abuse was similar. She found that behaviours which would be considered abusive (both physically and sexually) in North America were seen as part of the continuum of normal child rearing practices in Chile. Thus, although the scale could be translated from a linguistic point of view, its results would not have been valid in a different context.

The next step, one which is unfortunately frequently omitted, is called 'back-translation.' Another bilingual person, one who was not associated with the translation phase and again preferably knowledgeable, translates the new version back into English. If the meaning seems to have been lost or altered, then that item should go through the process again.

Once the translation is done, however, there is little assurance that the psychometric properties of the scale (i.e. its reliability and validity) have remained constant. It is therefore necessary to revalidate the instrument, as if it were a new one. For more information about the translating process, the reader should refer to Sechrest *et al.* (1972).

The question that therefore arises is whether translating a scale is worth the effort. It requires the translation itself, back translation, and then re-establishing the reliability and validity within the new context; in essence, exactly the same steps that are required for developing a new scale. The only difference is that the devising of new items has been replaced by the translating of old ones. Many scales have been translated, but problems still remain. For example, in two studies we have been involved in (O'Brien *et al.* 1994; Streiner *et al.* 1994) we used 'validated' versions of tests translated into French. The results, though, showed a lower incidence of migraine headaches in one study, and a higher self-reported quality of life in the other. The unresolved issue is whether these differences are due to cultural and other factors, or reflect subtle variations in the instruments used to measure them. Although questions may not have arisen had the prevalence rates been similar, there would still have been the issue of whether there actually are differences, but our translated instrument may have missed them.

The conclusion is that translating an instrument *can* be done, but it is as time-consuming as developing a new tool. Further, both similarities and differences in results must be interpreted with extreme caution.

References

Aaronson, N. K. (1988). Quantitative issues in health-related quality of life assessment. *Health Policy*, **10**, 217–30.

Aaronson, N. K. (1989). Quality of life assessment in clinical trials: Methodologic issues. *Controlled Clinical Trials*, **10**, 195S–208S.

Angleitner, A., John, O. P., and Löhr, F-J. (1986). It's *what* you ask and *how* you ask it: An itemmetric analysis of personality questionnaires. In *Personality assessment via questionnaires* (ed. A. Angleitner and J. S. Wiggins) pp. 61–107. Springer-Verlag, New York.

Aracena, M., Balladares, E., and Román, F. (1994). *Factores de riesgo para maltrato infantil, a nivel del sistema familiar: Una mirador cualitativa*. Documento de Trabajo N.1. Universidad de la Fronter, Temuco, Chile.

Becker, M. H., Maiman, L. A., Kirscht, J. P., Haefner, D. P., Drachman, R. H., and Taylor, D. W. (1979). Patient perception and compliance: Recent studies of the health belief model. In *Compliance in health care* (eds. R. B. Haynes and D. L. Sackett) pp. 78–109. Johns Hopkins University Press, Baltimore.

Bombardier, C., Ware, J., Russell, I. J., Larson, M., Chalmers, A., and Read, J. L. (1986). Auranofin therapy and quality of life in patients with rheumatoid arthritis: Results of a multicenter trial. *American Journal of Medicine*, **81**, 565–78.

Brumback, G. B., and Howell, M. A. (1972). Rating the clinical effectiveness of employed physicians. *Journal of Applied Psychology*, **56**, 241–4.

Cowles, J. T. and Kubany, A. J. (1959). Improving the measurement of clinical performance of medical students. *Journal of Clinical Psychology*, **15**, 139–42.

Cronbach, L. J. (1990). *Essentials of psychological testing* (5th edn.). Harper and Row, New York.

Feightner, J. W. (1985). Patient management problems. In *Assessing clinical competence* (eds. V. R. Neufeld and G. R. Norman) pp. 183–200). Springer-Verlag, New York.

Glass, G. V., McGaw, B., and Smith, M. L. (1981). *Meta-analysis in social research*. Sage, Beverly Hills, CA.

Goldberg, L. R. (1971). A historical survey of personality scales and inventories. In *Advances in psychological assessment*, Vol. 2 (ed. P. McReynolds) pp. 293–336. Science and Behavior, Palo Alto, CA.

Guyatt, G. H., Eagle, D. J., Sackett, B., Willan, A., Griffith, L., McIlroy, W., *et al.* (1993). Measuring quality of life in the frail elderly. *Journal of Clinical Epidemiology*, **46**, 1433–44.

Hathaway, S. R. and McKinley, J. C. (1951). *Manual for the Minnesota Multiphasic Personality Inventory* (rev.) Psychological Corporation, New York.

Kruis, W., Thieme, C., Weinzierl, M., Schuessler, P., Holl, J., and Paulus, W. (1984). A diagnostic score for the irritable bowel syndrome: Its value in the exclusion of organic disease. *Gastroenterology*, **87**, 1–7.

Liang, M. H., Larson, M. G., Cullen, K. E., and Schwartz, J. A. (1985). Comparative measurement efficiency and sensitivity of five health status instruments for arthritis research. *Arthritis and Rheumatism*, **28**, 542–7.

McFarlane, A. H., Norman, G. R., Streiner, D. L., Roy, R. G., and Scott, D. J. (1980). A longitudinal study of the influence of the psychosocial environment on health status: A preliminary report. *Journal of Health and Social Behavior*, **21**, 124–33.

McFarlane, A. H., Neale, K. A., Norman, G. R., Roy, R. G., and Streiner, D. L. (1981). Methodological issues in developing a scale to measure social support. *Schizophrenia Bulletin*, **7**, 90–100.

McHorney, C. A., Ware, J. E., Lu, J. F. R., and Sherbourne, C. D. (1994). The MOS 36-item Short Form health survey (SF–36): III. Tests of data quality, scaling assumptions, and reliability across diverse patient groups. *Medical Care*, **32**, 40–66.

Messick, S. (1980). Test validity and the ethics of assessment. *American Psychologist*, **35**, 1012–27.

Moos, R. H. (1984). *Menstrual distress questionnaire*. Stanford University Medical Center, Palo Alto, CA.

O'Brien, B., Goeree, R., and Streiner, D. L. (1994). Prevalence of migraine headache in Canada: A population-based survey. *International Journal of Epidemiology*, **23**, 1020–6.

Parkerson, G. R., Connis, R. T., Broadhead, W. E., Patrick, D. L. Taylor, T. R., and Tse, C. J. (1993). Disease-specific versus generic measurement of health-related quality of life in insulin-dependent diabetic patients. *Medical Care*, **31**, 629–39.

Patrick, D. L. and Deyo, R. A. (1989). Generic and disease-specific measures in assessing health status and quality of life. *Medical Care*, **27** (Supplement), S217–32.

Sechrest, L., Fay, T. L., and Hafeez Zaidi, S. M. (1972). Problems of translation in cross-cultural research. *Journal of Cross-Cultural Psychology*, **3**, 41–56.

Shannon, C. and Weaver, W. (1949). *The mathematical theory of communication*. University of Illinois Press, Urbana, IL.

Streiner, D. L., O'Brien, B., and Dean, D. (1994). *Quality of life in major depression: A comparison of instruments*. Paper presented at the 19th Annual Meeting of the Collegium Internationale Neuro-Psychopharmacologicum, Washington DC.

Taylor, J. A. (1953). A personality scale of manifest anxiety. *Journal of Abnormal and Social Psychology*, **48**, 285–90.

Taylor, S. J. and Bogden, R. (1984). *Introduction to qualitative research methods*. Wiley, New York.

Ullman, L. P. and Giovannoni, J. M. (1964). The development of a self-report measure of the process-reactive continuum. *Journal of Nervous and Mental Disease*, **138**, 38–42.

Wechsler, D. (1958). *The measurement and appraisal of adult intelligence* (4th edn). Williams and Wilkins, Baltimore.

Willms, D. G. and Johnson, N. A. (1993). *Essentials in qualitative research: A notebook for the field*. Unpublished manuscript.

4

Scaling responses

Introduction

Having devised a set of questions using the methods outlined in the previous chapter, we must choose a method by which responses will be obtained. The choice of method is dictated, at least in part, by the nature of the question asked. For example, a question like 'Have you ever gone to church?' leads fairly directly to a response method consisting of two boxes, one labelled 'Yes' and the other 'No'. By contrast, the question 'How religious are you?' does not dictate a simple two-category response, and a question like 'Do you believe that religious instruction leads to racial prejudice?' may require the use of more subtle and sophisticated techniques to obtain valid responses.

There has been a bewildering amount of research in this area, in disciplines ranging from psychology to economics. Often the results are conflicting, and the correct conclusions are frequently counter-intuitive. In this chapter, we describe a wide variety of scaling methods, indicate their appropriate use, and make recommendations regarding a choice of methods.

Some basic concepts

In considering approaches to the development of response scales, it is helpful to first consider the kinds of possible responses which may arise. A basic division is between those responses which are categorical, such as race, religion or marital status and those which are continuous variables like haemoglobin, blood pressure, or the amount of pain recorded on a 100 mm line. A second related feature of response scales is commonly referred to as the *level of measurement*. If the response consists of named categories, such as particular symptoms, a job classification, or religious denomination, the variable is called a *nominal* variable. Ordered categories, such as staging in breast cancer, educational level (less than high school, high school diploma, some college or university, university degree, postgraduate degree) are called *ordinal* variables. By contrast, variables in which the interval between responses and constant is known are called *interval* variables, naturally. Temperature, measured in degrees Celsius or Fahrenheit, is an interval variable. Generally speaking, rating scales, where the response is on a five-point or seven-point scale, are not considered interval level measurement,

---

Have you ever had a chest X-ray?   yes __ no __

Which of the following symptoms are you currently experiencing?

    Headaches __
    Dizziness __
    Cough   __
    Colds   __
    Other   (please write in) _____

Are you able to climb the stairs?   yes __ no __

I think that people are watching me.   true __ false __

Fig. 4.1 Examples of questions requiring categorical judgements.

since we can never be sure that the distance between 'strongly disagree' and 'disagree' is the same as between 'agree' and 'strongly agree'. However, some methods have been devised to achieve interval-level measurement with subjective scales, as will be discussed. Finally, variables where there is a meaningful zero point, so that the ratio of two responses has some meaning, are called *ratio* variables. Temperature measured in Kelvin is a ratio variable, temperature degrees in Fahrenheit or Celsius is not.

What is the significance of these distinctions? The important difference lies between nominal and ordinal data on one hand, and interval and ratio variables on the other. In the latter case, measures such as means, standard deviations, and differences among means can be interpreted and the broad class of techniques called 'parametric statistics' can therefore be used for analysis. By contrast, since it makes no sense to speak of the average religion or average sex of a sample of people, nominal and ordinal data must be considered as frequencies in individual categories, and 'non-parametric' statistics must be used for analysis. The distinction between these two types of analysis is described in any introductory statistics book, such as those listed in Appendix A.

Categorical judgements

One form of question frequently used in health sciences requires only a categorical judgement by the respondent, either as a 'yes–no' response, or as a simple check. The responses would then result in a *nominal* scale of measurement. Some examples are shown in Figure 4.1. Care must be taken to ensure that questions are written clearly and unambiguously, as discussed in Chapter 5. However, there is little difficulty in deciding on the appropriate response method.

Perhaps the most common error when using categorical questions is that they

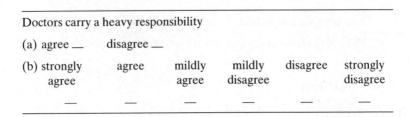

Fig. 4.2 Example of a continuous judgement.

are frequently employed in circumstances where the response is not, in fact, categorical. Attitudes and behaviours often lie on a continuum. When we ask a question like 'Do you have trouble climbing stairs?', we ignore the fact that there are varying degrees of trouble. Even the best athlete might have difficulty negotiating the stairs of a skyscraper at one run without some degree of discomfort. What we wish to find out presumably, is *how much* trouble the respondent has in negotiating an ordinary flight of stairs.

Ignoring the continuous nature of many responses leads to three difficulties. The first is fairly obvious: since different people may have different ideas about what constitutes a positive response to a question, there will likely be error introduced into the responses, as well as uncertainty and confusion on the part of respondents.

The second problem is perhaps more subtle. Even if all respondents have a similar conception of the category boundaries, there will still be error introduced into the measurement because of the limited choice of response levels. For example, the statement in Figure 4.2 might be responded to in one of two ways, as indicated in (a) and (b): the first method effectively reduces all positive opinions, ranging from strong to mild, to a single number, and similarly for all negative feelings. The effect is a potential loss of information and a corresponding reduction in reliability.

The third problem, which is a consequence of the second, is that dichotomizing a continuous variable leads to a loss of *efficiency* of the instrument, and a reduction in its correlation with other measures. A more efficient instrument requires fewer subjects in order to show an effect than a less efficient one. Suissa (1991) calculated that a dichotomous outcome is, at best, 67 per cent as efficient as a continuous one; depending on how the measure was dichotomized, this can drop to under 10 per cent. Under the best of circumstances, then, if you needed 67 subjects to show an effect when the outcome is measured along a continuum, you would need 100 subjects to demonstrate the same effect when the outcome is dichotomized. When circumstances are not as ideal, the inflation in required sample size can be 10 or more. Similarly, Hunter and Schmidt (1990) showed that if the dichotomy resulted in a 50–50 split, with half of the subjects in one group and half in the other, the correlation of that instrument with another is reduced by 20 per cent. Any other split results in a greater attenuation; if the result is that 10 per cent of the subjects are in one group and 90 per cent in the other, then the reduction is 41 per cent.

We have demonstrated this result with real data on several occasions. In a recent study of the certification examinations in internal medicine in Canada, the reliability of the original scores, inter-rater and test–retest, was 0.76 and 0.47 respectively. These scores were then converted to a pass–fail decision and the reliability recalculated. The comparable statistics for these decisions were 0.69 and 0.36, a loss of about 0.09 in reliability.

An even more dramatic demonstration of the phenomenon derives from a standardized clinical skills test called the Objective Structured Clinical Examination or OSCE (Harden and Gleeson 1979). In this examination, students are required to pass through a series of brief encounters with simulated patients, and perform circumscribed manoeuvres, such as auscultating a patient or taking a brief history of chest pain. The examiner is furnished with a standard checklist of required actions, and scores such as 'Done' versus 'Not Done', or alternatively, 'Done Well', 'Done Poorly', or 'Not Done' are assigned by observers. These scores are then summed to create a total score for the station. One appeal of the method is its apparent objectivity; however, several studies (van der Vleuten *et al.* 1991), comparing the summary score from the checklist to a single global rating on a 5 or 7 point scale, have shown that the global rating has consistently equal or better reliability than the checklist score, despite the fact that the latter may be based on 10 to 30 items, whereas the former is derived from a single score. The illusion of objectivity may not be reflected in reliability.

There are two common, but invalid, objections to the use of multiple response levels. The first is that the researcher is only interested in whether respondents agree or disagree, so it is not worth the extra effort. This argument confuses measurement with decision-making; the decision can always be made after the fact by establishing a cutoff point on the response continuum, but information lost from the original responses cannot be recaptured.

A second argument is that the additional categories are only adding noise or error to the data; people cannot make finer judgements than 'agree–disagree'. Although there may be particular circumstances where this is true, in general the evidence indicates that people are capable of much finer discriminations; this will be reviewed in a later section of the chapter where we discuss the appropriate number of response steps (p. 35).

Continuous judgements

Accepting that many of the variables of interest to health care researchers are continuous rather than categorical, methods must be devised to quantify these judgements.

The approaches which we will review fall into three broad categories: *direct estimation* techniques, in which subjects are required to indicate their response

---

How severe has your arthritic pain been today?

pain as   no
bad as it _____ pain
could be

Fig. 4.3 The visual analogue scale (VAS).

by a mark on a line or check in a box; *comparative* methods, in which subjects choose among a series of alternatives which have been previously calibrated by a separate criterion group; and *econometric* methods, in which the subjects describe their preference by anchoring it to extreme states (perfect health—death).

Direct estimation methods
Direct estimation methods are designed to elicit from the subject a direct quantitative estimate of the magnitude of an attribute. The approach is usually straightforward, as in the example used above, where we asked for a response on a six-point scale ranging from 'strongly agree' to 'strongly disagree'. This is one of many variations, although all share many common features. We begin by describing the main contenders, then we will explore their advantages and disadvantages.

Visual analogue scales
The visual analogue scale (VAS) is the essence of simplicity—a line of fixed length, usually 100 mm, with anchors like 'no pain' and 'pain as bad as it could be' at the extreme ends, and no words describing intermediate positions. An example is shown in Figure 4.3. Respondents are required to place a mark, usually an 'X' or a vertical line, on the line corresponding to their perceived state. The method has been used extensively in medicine to assess a variety of constructs; pain (Huskisson 1974), mood (Aitken 1969), and functional capacity (Scott and Huskisson 1978), among many others.

The VAS has also been used for the measurement of change (Scott and Huskisson 1979). In this approach, researchers are interested in perceptions of the degree to which patients feel they have improved as a result of treatment. The strategy used is to show patients, at the end of a course of treatment, where they had marked the line prior to commencing treatment, and then asking them to indicate, by a second line, their present state. There are a number of conceptual and methodological issues in the measurement of change, by VAS or other means, which will be addressed in Chapter 11.

Proponents are enthusiastic in their writings regarding the advantages of the method over its usual rival, a scale in which intermediate positions are labelled (e.g. 'mild', 'moderate', 'severe'); however, the authors frequently then demonstrate a substantial correlation between the two methods (Downie *et al.* 1978) suggesting that the advantages are more perceived than real. One also suspects that the method provides an illusion of precision, since a number given to two decimal places (e.g. a length measured in millimetres) has an apparent accuracy of 1 per cent. Of course, although one can measure a response to this degree of precision, there is no guarantee that the response accurately represents the underlying attribute to the same degree of resolution.

The simplicity of the VAS has contributed to its popularity, although there is some evidence that patients may not find it as simple and appealing as researchers; in one study described above (Huskisson 1974), 7 per cent of patients were unable to complete a VAS, as against 3 per cent for a graphic rating scale. Similarly, Bosi Ferraz *et al.* (1990) found that in Brazil, illiterate subjects had more difficulty with a VAS than with numerical or adjectival scales; their test–retest reliabilities, although statistically significant, were below an acceptable level. Some researchers in geriatrics have concluded that there may be an age effect in the perceived difficulty in using the VAS, leading to a modification of the technique. Instead of a horizontal line, they have used a vertical 'thermometer', which is apparently easier for older people to complete.

Perhaps the most serious problem with the VAS is not inherent in the scale at all. In many applications of the VAS in health sciences, the attribute of interest, such as pain, is assessed with a single scale, as in the example shown earlier. However, the reliability of a scale is directly related to the number of items in the scale, so that the one-item VAS test is likely to demonstrate low reliability in comparison to longer scales. The solution, of course, is to lengthen the scale by including multiple VASs, to assess related aspects of the attribute of interest.

In conclusion, although the VAS approach has the merit of simplicity, there appears to be sufficient evidence that other methods may yield more precise measurement, and possibly increased levels of satisfaction among respondents.

Adjectival scales
In contrast to the research on the VAS, most investigations in psychological rating scales have focused on scales with adjectival descriptions and discrete or continuous responses. Examples of the two approaches are shown in Figure 4.4.

It is evident that the rating scale with continuous responses bears close resemblance to the VAS, with the exception that additional descriptions are introduced at intermediate positions. Although proponents of the VAS eschew the use of descriptors, an opposite position is taken by psychometricians regarding rating scales. Guilford (1954) states 'nothing should be left undone to give the rater a clear, unequivocal conception of the continuum along which he is to evaluate objects . . . '(p. 292).

Specific scaling methods
Within this broad class of rating scales, there are several specific formats which have achieved wide popularity. One is the *Likert scale* (Likert 1952), in which the rater expresses an opinion by rating his agreement with a series of statements

(a) Discrete responses

What is the student's history-taking ability?

much below   below   average   above   much above
  average   average   average   average

☐   ☐   ☐   ☐   ☐

(b) Continuous responses

The physician's interpersonal manners were:

most   unpleasant neutral   pleasant   most
unpleasant   pleasant

Fig. 4.4 Examples of adjectival scales.

The world is in danger of nuclear holocaust.

strongly   agree   no opinion   disagree   strongly
agree   disagree

Fig. 4.5 Examples of a Likert scale.

MY ILLNESS

painful   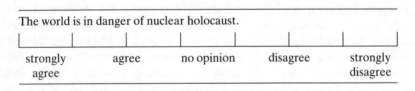   painless

embarrassing   not embarrassing

serious   mild

Fig. 4.6 The semantic differential scale.

like Figure 4.5. The only unique characteristic of the Likert scale is that responses are framed on an agree–disagree continuum.

A second standard approach, the *semantic differential scale* (Osgood *et al.* 1957), is used to obtain ratings of a particular object on a series of dimensions, as shown in Figure 4.6. The basic notion is to define a number of related dimensions of a characteristic on a series of continuous bipolar scales.

General issues in the construction of continuous scales

Regardless of the specific approach adopted, there are a number of questions which must be addressed in designing a rating scale to maximize precision and minimize bias.

1. *How many steps should there be?* The choice of the number of steps or boxes on a scale is not primarily an aesthetic issue. We indicated earlier in the discussion of categorical ratings that the use of two categories to express an underlying continuum will result in a loss of information. The argument can be extended to the present circumstances; if the number of levels is less than the rater's ability to discriminate, the result will be a loss of information.

Although the ability to discriminate would appear to be highly contingent on the particular situation, there is evidence that this is not the case. A number of studies have shown that for reliability coefficients in the range normally encountered, from 0.4 to 0.9, the reliability drops as fewer categories are used. Nishisato and Torii (1970) studied this empirically by generating distributions of two variables with known correlations, ranging from 0.1 to 0.9 in steps of 0.2. They then rounded off the numbers as if they were creating a scale of a particular number of steps. For example, if the original numbers fell in the range from 1.000 to 10.000, a two-point scale was created by calling any number less than 5.000 a 0, and any number greater than or equal to 5.000 a 1. A ten-point scale was created by rounding off up to the decimal point, resulting in discrete values ranging from 1 to 10. The final step in this simulation was to recalculate the correlation using the rounded numbers. Since the rounding process resulted in the loss of precision, this should have the effect of reducing the correlation between the sets of numbers. The original correlation corresponds to the test–retest reliability of the original data, and the recalculated correlation, using the rounded-off numbers is equivalent to the reliability which would result from a scale with 2, 5 or 10 boxes, with everything else held constant.

As can be seen from Figure 4.7, the loss in reliability for 7 and 10 categories is quite small. However, the use of five categories reduces the reliability by about 12 per cent, and the use of only two categories results in an average reduction of the reliability coefficient of 35 per cent. These results were confirmed by other studies, and suggest that the minimum number of categories used by raters should be in the region of five to seven. Of course, a common problem of ratings is that raters seldom use the extreme positions on the scale, and this should be taken into account when designing the scale, as discussed in Chapter 6.

2. *Is there a maximum number of categories?* From a purely statistical perspective, the answer is 'no', since the actual reliability approaches the theoretical maximum asymptotically.

However, there is good evidence that, in a wide variety of tasks, people are unable to discriminate much beyond seven levels. In a now-classic article entitled 'The magic number seven plus or minus two: Some limits on our capacity for processing information', Miller (1956) showed that the limit of short-term memory is of the order of seven 'chunks' (hence seven digit tele-

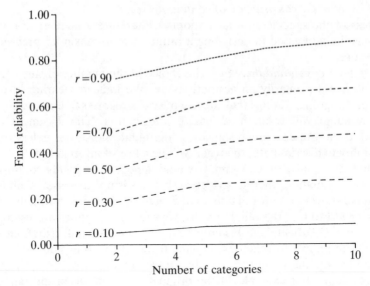

Fig. 4.7 The effect of the number of scale categories on reliability.

phone numbers). Interestingly, the first two-thirds of the article are devoted to discussion of discrimination judgements. In an impressive number of situations, such as judging the pitch or loudness of a sound, the saltiness of a solution, the position of a point on a line, or the size of a square, the upper limit of the number of categories which could be discriminated was remarkably near seven (plus or minus two).

There is certainly no reason to presume that people will do any better in judgements of sadness, pain, or interpersonal skill. Thus it is reasonable to presume that the upper practical limit of useful levels on a scale, taking into account human foibles, can be set at seven. Certainly these findings clearly suggest that the 'one in a hundred' precision of the VAS is illusory; people are probably mentally dividing it into about seven segments.

There are two caveats to this recommendation. First, recognizing the common 'end-aversion bias' described in Chapter 6, where people tend to avoid the two extremes of a scale, there may be some advantage to designing nine levels on the scale. Conversely, when a large number of individual items are designed to be summed to a create a scale score, it is likely that reducing the number of levels to five or three will not result in significant loss of information.

3. *Should there be an even or odd number of categories?* Where the response scale is unipolar, that is to say, scale values range from zero to a maximum, then the question is of little consequence, and can be decided on stylistic grounds. However for bipolar scales (like strongly agree—strongly disagree) the provision of an odd number of categories allows raters the choice of expressing no opinion. Conversely, an even number of boxes forces the raters to commit themselves to

one side or the other. There is no absolute rule; depending on the needs of the particular research it may or may not be desirable to allow a neutral position.

4. *Should all the points on the scale be labelled, or only the ends?* Most of the research indicates that there is relatively little difference between scales with adjectives under each box and end-anchored scales (e.g. Dixon *et al*. 1984; Newstead and Arnold 1989). In fact, subjects seem to be more influenced by the adjectives on the ends of the scales than those in the intermediate positions (e.g. Frisbie and Brandenburg 1979; Wildt and Mazis 1978). There is some tendency for end-anchored scales to pull responses to the ends, producing greater variability. Similarly, if only every other box is defined (usually because the scale constructor cannot think of enough adjectives), the labelled boxes tend to be endorsed more often than the unlabelled ones.

5. *Do the adjectives always convey the same meaning?* Many adjectival scales use words or phrases like 'almost always', 'often', 'seldom', or 'rarely' in order to elicit judgements about the frequency of occurrence of an event or the intensity of a feeling. The question that arises from this is: to what extent do people agree on the meanings associated with these adjectives? Most research regarding agreement has focused on people's estimations of probabilities which they assign to words like 'highly probable' or 'unlikely', and the data are not encouraging. The estimated probability of a 'highly probable' event ranged from 0.60 to 0.99. Other phrases yielded even more variability: 'usually' went from 0.15 to 0.99, 'rather unlikely' from 0.01 to 0.75, and 'cannot be excluded' from 0.07 to 0.98 (Lichtenstein and Newman 1967; Bryant and Norman 1980). Part of the problem is the vagueness of the terms themselves. Another difficulty is that the meanings assigned to adjectives differ with the context. For example, the term 'often' connotes a higher absolute frequency for common events as opposed to rare ones; and 'not too often' carries different meanings depending on whether the activity described is an exciting or a boring one (Schaeffer 1991).

6. *Do numbers placed under the boxes influence the responses?* Some adjectival scales also put numbers under the words, to help the respondent find an appropriate place along the line. Does it matter whether the numbers range from 1 to 7 or from −3 to +3? What little evidence exists suggests that the answer is 'yes'. Schwarz *et al*. (1991) gave subjects a scale consisting of a series of 11-point Likert scales. In all cases, one extreme was labelled 'not at all successful' and the other end 'extremely successful'. However, for some subjects, the numbers under the adjectives went from −5 to +5, while for others they went from 0 to 10. Although the questionnaire was completed anonymously, minimizing the chances that the respondents would attempt to present themselves well to the examiner (see *social desirability* bias in Chapter 6), the numbers made a large difference. When only positive integers were used, 34 per cent of the subjects used the lower (relatively unsuccessful) half of the scale (0 to 5), and had a mean value of 5.96. However, when the −5 to +5 numbering scheme was used, only 13 per cent used the lower half, and the mean value was pushed up to 7.38. Thus, it appeared as if the subjects were using the numbers to help them interpret the

meaning of the adjectives, and that the negative scale values conveyed a differ-ent meaning from the positive ones.

7. *Should the order of successive question responses change?* Some scales reverse the order of responses at random, so that successive questions may have response categories which go from low to high or high to low, in order to avoid 'yea-saying' bias (discussed in Chapter 6). The dilemma is that a careless subject may not notice the change, resulting in almost totally uninterpretable responses. Of course, with reversed order, the researcher will *know* that the responses are uninterpretable due to carelessness, whereas if order is not reversed the subject looks consistent whether or not he paid attention to individual questions.

8. *Can it be assumed that the data are interval?* As we indicated earlier, one issue regarding the use of rating scales is that they are, strictly speaking, on an ordinal level of measurement. Although responses are routinely assigned numerical values, so that 'strongly agree' becomes a 7 and 'strongly disagree' becomes a 1, we really have no guarantee that the true distance between successive categories is the same; i.e. that the distance between 'strongly agree' and 'agree' is really the same as the distance between 'strongly disagree' and 'disagree'. The matter is of more than theoretical interest, since the statistical methods which are used to analyse the data, such as analysis of variance, rest on this assumption of equality of distance. Considerable debate has surrounded the dangers inherent in the assumption of interval properties. The arguments range from the extreme position that the numbers themselves are interval (e.g. 1, 2, . . . , 7) and can be manipulated as interval-level data regardless of their relationship to the underly-ing property being assessed (Gaito 1982) to the opposite view that the numbers must be demonstrated to have a linear relationship with the underlying property before interval-level measurement can be assumed (Townsend and Ashby 1984). The debate shows no sign of resolution. Nevertheless, from a pragmatic view-point, it appears that under most circumstances, unless the distribution of scores is severely skewed, one can analyse data from rating scales as if they were inter-val without introducing severe bias.

Spector (1976) attempted to use a variation of Thurstone scaling in order to assign interval scale values to a variety of adjectives. He came up with three lists of categories: evaluation (consisting of words such as 'terrible', 'unsatisfactory', and 'excellent'); agreement (e.g. 'slightly', 'moderately', 'very much'); and fre-quency ('rarely' through 'most of the time'). Each list contains 13 words or phrases, allowing the scale constructor to select five or seven with equal inter-vals. While these lists may help in rank ordering the adjectives, Spector unfortu-nately did not provide any indices of the agreement among the judges.

Critique of direct estimation methods
Direct estimation methods, in various forms, are pervasive in research involving subjective judgements. They are relatively easy to design, require little pre-test-ing in contrast to the comparative methods described next, and are easily under-stood by subjects. Nevertheless, the ease of design and administration is both an

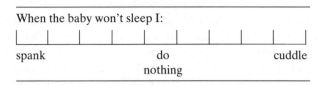

Fig. 4.8 Likert scaling of a question about child abuse.

asset and a liability: because the intent of questions framed on a rating scale is often obvious to both researcher and respondent, bias in response can result. The issue of bias is covered in more detail in Chapter 6; but we mention some problems briefly here. One bias of rating scales is the *halo effect*; since items are frequently ordered in a single column on a page it is possible to rapidly rate all items on the basis of a global impression, paying little attention to the individual categories. People also rarely commit themselves to the extreme categories on the scale, effectively reducing the precision of measurement. Finally, it is common in ratings of other people, staff or students, to have a strong positive skew, so that the average individual is rated well above average, again sacrificing precision.

In choosing among specific methods, the scaling methods we have described differ for historical rather than substantive reasons, and it is easy to find examples which have features of more than one approach. The important point is to follow the general guidelines: specific descriptors, seven or more steps, and so forth, rather than becoming preoccupied with choosing among alternatives.

Comparative methods

Although rating scales have a number of advantages—simplicity, ease and speed of completion—there are occasions where their simplicity would be a deterrent to acquiring useful data. For example, in a study of predictors of child abuse (Shearman *et al*. 1983), one scale questioned parents on the ways they handled irritating child behaviours. A number of infant behaviours were presented, and parents were to specify how they dealt with each problem. Casting this scale into a rating format (which was not done) might result in items like those in Figure 4.8.

The ordered nature of the response scale would make it unlikely that parents would place any marks to the left of the neutral position. Instead, we would like the respondent to simply indicate her likely action, or select it from a list. If we could then assign a value to each behaviour, we could generate a score for the respondent based on the sum of the assigned values.

The approach which was used was one of a class of *comparative* methods, called the *paired-comparison* technique, whereby respondents were simply asked to indicate which behaviour—'punish', 'cuddle', 'hit', 'ignore', 'put in room'—they were likely to do in a particular circumstance. These individual responses were assigned a numerical value in advance on the basis of a survey of a group of experts (in this case day-care workers), who had been asked to compare each parental response to a situation to all other possible responses, and select the most appropriate response for each of these pairwise comparisons.

The comparative methods also address a general problem with all rating scales, the ordinal nature of the scale. Comparative methods circumvent the difficulty by directly scaling the value of each description before obtaining responses, to ensure that the response values are on an interval scale.

There are three comparative methods commonly used in the literature: *Thurstone's method* of equal-appearing intervals, *Guttman scaling*, and the *paired-comparison* technique. Each is discussed below.

Thurstone's method of equal-appearing intervals

The method begins with the selection of 100–200 statements relevant to the topic about which attitudes are to be assessed. Following the usual approaches to item generation, these statements are edited to be short and to the point. Each statement is then typed on a separate card, and a number of judges are asked to sort them into a single pile from the lowest or least desirable to highest. Extreme anchor statements, at the opposite ends of the scale, may be provided. Following the completion of this task by a large number of judges, the median rank of each statement is computed, which then becomes the scale value for each statement.

As an example, if we were assessing attitude to doctors, we might assemble a large number of statements like 'I will always do anything my doctor prescribes', 'I think doctors are overpaid', and 'Most doctors are aware of their patients' feelings'. Suppose we gave these statements to nine judges (actually, many more would be necessary for stable estimates) and the statement 'I think nurses provide as good care as doctors' was ranked respectively by the nine judges 17, 18, 23, 25, 26, 27, 28, 31, and 35, of 100 statements. The median rank of this statement is the rank of the fifth person, in this case 26, so this would be the value assigned to the statement.

The next step in the procedure is to select a limited number of statements, about 25 in number, in such a manner that the intervals between successive items are about equal and they span the entire range of values. These items then comprise the actual scale.

Finally, in applying the scale to an individual, the respondent is asked to indicate which statements apply to him/her. The respondents' score is then calculated as the average score of items selected.

Paired comparison technique

The paired-comparison method is directed at similar goals, and uses a similar approach to the Thurstone method. In both methods, the initial step is to calibrate a limited set of items so that they can be placed on an interval scale. Subjects' responses to these items are then used in developing a score by simply

Table 4.1 *Probability of selecting each behaviour over others*

Behaviour	1 Punish	2 Spank	3 Ignore	4 Cuddle
1. Punish	0.50	0.60	0.70	0.90
2. Spank	0.40	0.50	0.70	0.80
3. Ignore	0.30	0.30	0.50	0.70
4. Cuddle	0.10	0.20	0.30	0.50

summing or averaging the calibration weights of those items endorsed by a subject.

Where the two methods differ is in their approach to calibration. Thurstone scaling begins with a large number of items, and asks people to judge each item against all others by explicitly ranking the items. By contrast, the paired-comparison method, as the name implies, asks judges to explicitly compare each item one at a time to each of the remaining items, and simply judge which of the two has more of the property under study. Considering the example which began this chapter, our child care workers would be asked to indicate the more desirable parental behaviour in pairwise fashion as follows:

punish—spank

punish—cuddle

punish—ignore

spank —cuddle

spank —ignore

cuddle—ignore

In actual practice, a larger sample of parental behaviours would be used, order from right to left would be randomized, and the order of presentation of the cards would be randomized.

If such a list of choices were given to a series of ten judges, the data would be then displayed as in Table 4.1, indicating the proportion of times each alternative was chosen over each other option.

Reading down the first column, the table shows, for example that 'punish' was chosen over 'spank' by 40 per cent of the subjects. Note that the diagonal entries are assumed equal to 0.50, i.e. 'punish' is selected over 'punish' 50 per cent of the time; also, the top right values are the 'mirror image' of those in the bottom left.

The next step is to use the property of the normal curve to convert this table to z-values. This bit of sleight-of-hand is best illustrated by reference to Figure 4.9, which shows the 40 per cent point on a normal curve; that is, the point on the curve where 40 per cent of the distribution falls to the left. If the mean of the

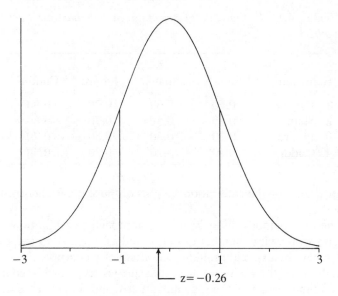

Fig. 4.9 The normal curve.

Table 4.2 *z-values of the probabilities*

Behaviour	1	2	3	4
1. Punish	0.00	0.26	0.53	1.28
2. Spank	−0.26	0.00	0.53	0.85
3. Ignore	−0.53	−0.53	0.00	0.53
4. Cuddle	−1.28	−0.85	−0.53	0.00
Total z	−2.07	−1.12	+0.53	+2.66
Average z	−0.52	−0.28	+0.13	+0.66

curve is set to zero, and the standard deviation to 1, this occurs at a value of −0.26. As a result, the probability value of 0.40 is replaced by a z-value of −0.26. In practice, these values are determined by consulting a table of the normal curve in any statistical text. The resulting values are shown in Table 4.2.

The z scores for each column are then summed and averaged, yielding the z score equivalent to the average probability of each item being selected over all other items. The resulting z score for 'punish' now becomes −0.52, and for 'cuddle' it is +0.66. The range of negative and positive numbers is a bit awkward, so a constant is often added to all the values to avoid negative weights. These weights can be assumed to have interval properties.

Table 4.3   *Guttman scaling*

I am able to:	Subject				
	A	B	C	D	E
Walk across the room	1	1	1	1	1
Climb the stairs	1	1	1	1	0
Walk one block outdoors	1	1	0	0	0
Walk more than one mile	1	0	0	0	0

All this manipulation is directed to the assignment of weights to each option. To use these weights for scoring a subject is straightforward; the score is simply the weight assigned to the option selected by the subject. If the questionnaire is designed in such a way that a subject may endorse multiple-response options, for example by responding to various infant behaviours like crying, not going to sleep, refusing to eat, the weights for all responses can be added or averaged since they are interval level measurements.

The Guttman method

The Guttman method begins, as does the Thurstone method, with a large sample of items. However, this is reduced by judgement of the investigator to a relatively small sample of 10–20 items which are thought to span the range of the attitude or behaviour assessed. As we shall see, in Guttman scaling, it is crucial that the items address only a single underlying attribute, since an individual score arises from the accumulated performance on all items.

These items are then administered directly to a sample of subjects, who are asked to endorse those items applicable to them. Unlike the alternative methods discussed in this section, there is no separate calibration step. The items are then tentatively ranked according to increasing amount of the attribute assessed, and responses are displayed in a subject-by-item matrix, with 1's indicating those items endorsed by a subject and 0's indicating the remaining items.

As an example, suppose we were assessing function of the lower limbs in a sample of people with osteo-arthritis. A display of the responses of five subjects to the following four items might resemble Table 4.3.

In this example, subject A gets a score of 4, subject B a score of 3, C and D attain scores of 2, and subject E a score of 1. This is an idealized example, since no 'reversals' occur, in which a subject endorsed a more difficult item (e.g. walk more than a mile) but not an easier one (e.g. climb the stairs). In reality, such reversals do occur, detracting from the strict ordering of the items implied by the method. There are a number of indices which reflect how much an actual scale deviates from perfect cumulativeness, of which the two most important are the *coefficient of reproducibility* and the *coefficient of scalability*.

The first, reproducibility, indicates the degree to which a person's scale score is a predictor of his or her response pattern. To calculate it, we must know the total number of subjects (N), the number for whom there was some error in the ordering (n_e), and the number of items (I). The coefficient is then:

$$Reproducibility = 1 - \frac{n_e}{I \times N}$$

If we gave our four-item scale to 150 people, and found that the order was correct for 109 cases and incorrect for 41, then the coefficient in this case would be:

$$1 - \frac{41}{150 \times 4} = 0.932$$

Reproducibility can vary between 0 and 1, and should be higher than 0.9 for the scale to be valid.

The coefficient of scalability reflects whether the scale is truly unidimensional and cumulative. Its calculation is complex and best left to computer programs. It, too, varies between 0 and 1, and should be at least 0.6.

Guttman scaling is best suited to behaviours which are developmentally determined (e.g. crawling, standing, walking, running), where mastery of one behaviour virtually guarantees mastery of lower-order behaviours. Thus it is useful in assessing development in children, decline due to progressively deteriorating disease, functional ability, and the like. It is *not* appropriate in assessing the kind of loss in function due to focal lesions that arises in stroke patients, where impairment of some function may be unrelated to impairment of other functions. Unlike the other methods discussed in this section, Guttman scales are unlikely to have interval scale properties.

Guttman scaling is also the basis of *latent-trait theory* (discussed in Chapter 12), which has emerged as a very powerful scaling method, and begins with a similar assumption of ordering of item difficulty and candidate ability. However, in contrast to Guttman scaling, latent-trait scaling explicitly assigns values to both items and subjects on an interval scale, and also deals successfully with the random processes which might result in departures from strict ordering demanded by the Guttman scale.

Critique of comparative methods
It is clear that any of the three comparative methods we have described requires considerably more time for development than any of the direct scaling methods. Nevertheless, this investment may be worthwhile under two circumstances. If it is desirable to disguise the ordinal property of the responses, as in the child abuse example, then the additional resources may be well spent. Secondly, the

Thurstone and paired-comparison methods guarantee interval-level measurement, which may be important in some applications, particularly when there are relatively few items in the scale.

With regard to choice among the methods, as we have indicated, the Guttman method has several disadvantages in comparison to other methods. It is difficult to select items with Guttman properties, and the scale has only ordinal properties. The choice between Thurstone and paired-comparison is more difficult. However, the Thurstone method is more practical when there are a large number of items desired in the scale, since the number of comparisons needed in the paired-comparison technique is roughly proportional to the square of the number of items.

Goal attainment scaling

Goal attainment scaling (GAS) is an attempt to construct scales which are tailored to specific individuals, yet can yield results which are measured on a common, ratio scale across all people. It got its start in the area of program evaluation (Kiresuk and Sherman 1968), but has been widely applied in clinical settings (e.g. Santa-Barbara *et al.* 1974; Stolee *et al.* 1992), where the criteria for 'success' may vary from one patient to another.

The heart of GAS is the 'goal attainment follow-up guide', which is a matrix having a series of goals across the top, and five levels down the left side. For each individual, three to five goals are identified; the number of goals need not be the same for all people. The five levels are comparable to a Likert scale, ranging from the 'most favourable outcome thought likely' (given a score of +2) to the 'least favourable outcome thought likely' (a score of −2), with the mid-point labelled 'expected level of success' (a score of 0). Within each box of the matrix are written the criteria for determining whether or not that level of outcome for the specific goal has been attained for the person. Since good research technique demands that outcome evaluation be done by a rater who is blind with respect to which group a subject is in, the criteria must be written in terms of concrete, observable outcomes. For example, if one of the goals for a subject in a geriatric reactivation program is 'meal preparation', then an expected level of success (a score of 0) may be 'Has cooked her own supper every night for the past week'. The most favourable outcome (+2) may be 'Has cooked all her meals for the past week', and the criterion for a score of +1 may be 'Has cooked all suppers and some of the other meals during the past week'. Conversely, the least favourable outcome (−2) could be that the person has not cooked at all, and a score of −1 is given if some cooking was done, but not every night.

There are three points to note. First, if the intervention works as intended, the experimental subjects should score 0 for all goals; a higher mean score for all people probably indicates that the goals were set too low, not that the program was wildly successful. Second, the criteria may vary from one person to the next; what is an 'expected level of success' for one individual may be somewhat favourable for a second, and least favourable for a third. The last point is that not all subjects need have the same goals.

After the goals have been selected, they can each be given a weight (which traditionally ranges between 1 and 9), reflecting the importance of that goal relative to the others. To compensate for the fact that people may have a different number of goals, and to make the final score have a mean of 50 with an SD of 10, the GAS score is calculated using the equation:

$$GAS = 50 + \frac{10 \; \Sigma \; w_i \, x_i}{\sqrt{(1 - r) \; \Sigma w_i^2 + r \; (\Sigma w_i)^2}}$$

where x_i is the score for scale i,
   w_i is the weight for scale i, and
   r is the average correlation among the scales.

The major advantage of GAS is its ability to tailor the scale to the specific goals of the individuals. However, this can also be one of its major limitations. Each subject has his or her own scale, with different numbers of goals, and varying criteria for each one. At the end of the study, it is possible to state that the intervention worked or did not work, but much more difficult to say where it did well and where it did poorly; poor scores on some scales may reflect more a bad choice of goals or criteria rather than a failure of the program. Moreover, comparisons across studies, and especially of different varieties of the intervention (e.g. various types of anti-inflammatory agents) become nearly impossible, since all successful trials will, by definition, have a mean of 50 and an SD of 10; less 'powerful' interventions will simply set more lenient criteria for success.

A second limitation of the technique is that it is extremely labour intensive. The clinicians or researchers must be taught how to formulate goals, and write criteria in objective, observable terms. Then, the raters have to be trained and tested to ensure that they reach adequate levels of reliability in scoring the goals. Thus, it seems as if GAS is potentially useful when (a) the objective is to evaluate an intervention as a whole, without regard to *why* it may work, or in comparing it to any other program; (b) the goals for each person are different; and (c) there are adequate resources for training goal setters and raters.

Econometric methods

The final class of scaling methods we will consider has its roots in a different discipline, economics, and has become increasingly popular in the medical literature in applications ranging from clinical trials to decision analysis. The problem for which these methods were devised involves assigning a numerical value to various health states. This arises in economics and health in the course of conducting cost/benefit studies, where it becomes necessary to scale benefits along a numerical scale so that cost/benefit ratios can be determined.

Note that economists are generally not interested in a specific individual's choice, but rather tend to obtain ratings of health states by averaging judgements from a large number of individuals in order to create a utility score for the state. Thus the focus of measurement is the described health state, not the characteristic of the individual respondent. This creates interesting problems for the assessment of reliability, which are explicitly dealt with in Chapter 9.

For example, consider a clinical trial comparing medical management of angina to coronary bypass surgery. Surgery offers a potential benefit in quality of life, but the trade-off is the finite possibility that the patient may not survive the operation or immediate post-operative period. How, then, does one make a rational choice between the two alternatives?

The first approach to the problem was developed in the 1950s, and is called the *Von Neumann–Morgenstern standard gamble* (1953). The subject is asked to consider the following scenario:

'You have been suffering from "angina" for several years. As a result of your illness, you experience severe chest pain after even minor physical exertion such as climbing stairs, or walking one block in cold weather. You have been forced to quit your job, and spend most days at home watching TV. Imagine that you are offered a possibility of an operation that will result in complete recovery from your illness. However, the operation carries some risk. Specifically, there is a probability "p" that you will die during the course of the operation. How large must "p" be before you will decline the operation and choose to remain in your present state?'

Clearly, the closer the present state is to perfect health, the smaller the risk of death one would be willing to entertain. Having obtained an estimate of 'p' from subjects, the value of the present state can be directly converted to a 0–1 scale by simply subtracting 'p' from 1, so that a tolerable risk of 1 per cent results in a value (called a 'utility') of 0.99 for the present state, and a risk of 50 per cent results in a utility of 0.50.

One difficulty with the 'standard gamble' is that few people, aside from statisticians and professional gamblers, are accustomed to dealing in probabilities. In order to deal with this problem, a number of devices are used to simplify the task. Subjects may be offered specific probabilities; e.g. 10 per cent chance of perioperative death, and 90 per cent chance of complete recovery, until they reach a point of indifference between the two alternatives. Visual aids, such as 'probability wheels', have also been used.

This difficulty in handling probabilities led to the development of an alternative method, called the *time tradeoff technique* (Torrance *et al.* 1972), which avoids the use of probabilities. One begins by estimating the likely remaining years of life for a healthy subject, using actuarial tables; i.e. if the patient is 30 years old we could estimate that he has about 40 years remaining. The previous question would then be rephrased as follows:

'Imagine living the remainder of your natural lifespan (40 years) in your present state. Contrast this with the alternative that you can return to perfect health for fewer years. How many years would you sacrifice if you could have perfect health?'

In practice, the respondent is presented with the alternatives of 40 years in her present state versus 0 years of complete health. The upper limit is decreased, and the lower limit increased, until a point of indifference is reached. The more years a subject is willing to sacrifice in exchange for a return to perfect health, presumably the worse he perceives his present health. The response (call it Y) can be converted to a scaled utility by the simple formula

$$U = (40 - Y)/40.$$

A thorough example of the application of this method in a clinical trial of support for relatives of demented elderly is given in Mohide *et al.* (1988).

Critique of econometric methods
We have presented the two methods as a means to measure individual health states. Although they are limited to the measurement of health states, they have been used both with real patients and with normal, healthy individuals imagining themselves to be ill.

The methods are quite difficult to administer and require a trained interviewer, so it remains to see whether they possess advantages over simpler techniques. One straightforward alternative would be a direct estimation of health state, using an adjectival or visual analogue scale. Torrance (1976) has shown that the time tradeoff and standard gamble methods yield similar results, which differed from the direct estimation method, suggesting that these methods may indeed be a more accurate reflection of the underlying state.

However, the methods are based on the notion that people make rational choices under conditions of uncertainty. There is an accumulation of evidence, reviewed in Chapter 6, which suggests that responses on rating scales can be influenced by a variety of extraneous factors. The methods reviewed in this section are no more immune to seemingly irrational behaviour, as reviewed by Llewellyn-Thomas and Sutherland (1986). As one example, framing a question in terms of 40 per cent survival instead of 60 per cent mortality will result in a shift of values. The problem addressed by the econometric methods assumed that context-free values could be elicited. It seems abundantly clear that such 'value-free' values are illusory, and a deeper understanding of the psychological variables which influence decisions and choices is necessary. Moreover, it appears that real patients assign higher (more positive) utilities to states of ill health than do normals imagining themselves in that state, casting doubt on the analogue studies. Last, the lower anchor is usually assumed to be death. There has been little work to examine conditions which some people (for example, Richard Dreyfuss in the movie *Whose Life Is It Anyway*) see as worse than death.

Multidimensional scaling

In the previous sections of this chapter, we discussed various techniques for creating scales which differentiate attributes along one dimension, such as a Guttman scale which taps mobility. However, there are situations in which we are interested in examining the similarities of different 'objects' which may vary along a number of separate dimensions. These objects can be diagnoses, occupations, social interactions, stressful life events, pain experiences, countries, faces, or almost anything else we can imagine (Weinberg 1991). The dimensions themselves are revealed by the analysis; that is, they are 'hidden' or 'latent', in that they are not directly observable from the data but inferred from the patterns that emerge in the way the objects group together. (For a more complete description of latent variables, see the chapter on Factor Analysis in Norman and Streiner (1994).) The family of techniques for performing this type of analysis is called *multidimensional scaling* (MDS). Very briefly, MDS begins with some index of how 'close' each object is to every other object, and then tries to determine how many dimensions underlie these evaluations of closeness.

To illustrate the technique, imagine that we want to determine what dimensions may underlie the similarities or differences among nine symptoms experienced by patients with various types of depression. The first step is to construct a *similarity matrix* (also called a *proximity matrix*). This can be done in a number of different ways. First, patients or clinicians can be given all possible pairs of symptoms, as with the paired comparison technique. But now, rather than choosing one or the other, they would indicate how similar the two symptoms are on, say, a 10-point scale, with 1 meaning not at all similar to 10 meaning most similar. Another way of constructing the matrix is to determine the frequency with which the symptoms co-occur in a sample of patients. A third method may be to ask patients to rate the perceived severity of each of the nine symptoms on some form of scale, and then correlate each symptom with all of the others. The mathematics of MDS do not care how the similarity matrix is formed—rating or judgements, frequency of co-occurrence, correlations, or any one of a number of other techniques. The difference shows up only in terms of how we interpret the results.

For the purposes of this example, let us assume that we used the frequency of co-occurrence, and obtained the results shown in Table 4.4. A score of 1 means that the symptoms always occur together, and 0 indicates that they never occur together. As would be expected, the maximum coefficient occurs along the main diagonal; sadness is more related to itself than to any other symptom. Conversely, coefficients of 0 reflect mutually exclusive symptoms, such as insomnia and hypersomnia.

MDS uses this matrix to determine the number of dimensions which underlie the similarities among the symptoms. There are a number of different computer programs which do this. They vary according to various assumptions which are made: whether the objects are differentiated holistically or in terms of separate attributes; and whether the proximities among the objects are measured on an ordinal or an interval scale. A description of the programs is given in an article by Weinberg (1991) and a monograph by Kruskal and Wish (1978). Irrespective of which program is used, the results are usually displayed in a graph, with each

Table 4.4 *Similarity matrix of nine symptoms of depression*

	A	B	C	D	E	F	G	H	I
A	1.00								
B	0.865	1.00							
C	0.495	0.691	1.00						
D	0.600	0.823	0.612	1.00					
E	0.125	0.135	0.402	0.127	1.00				
F	0.201	0.129	0.103	0.111	0.000	1.00			
G	0.125	0.581	0.513	0.578	0.713	0.399	1.00		
H	0.312	0.492	0.192	0.487	0.303	0.785	0.000	1.00	
I	0.105	0.223	0.332	0.201	0.592	0.762	0.414	0.185	1.00

A = Feeling of sadness
B = Pessimism
C = Decreased libido
D = Suicidal ideation
E = Weight gain
F = Weight loss
G = Hypersomnia
H = Early morning wakening
I = Psychomotor retardation

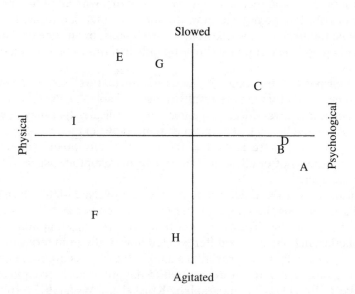

Fig. 4.10 Scatter plot of the results of MDS.

axis representing one dimension. The researcher then tries to determine what the dimensions represent, in terms of the underlying properties of the objects. For example, assume that the similarity matrix yielded just two interpretable dimensions. We can then plot the location of each symptom along these two dimensions, as in Figure 4.10.

The closer the symptoms are on the graph, the more similar they are to one another. It would appear as if the first dimension is differentiating symptoms which are primarily psychological from those which are more physiological in nature, while the second dimension reflects a continuum of psychomotor retardation versus agitation.

Most researchers stop at this point, and are content to have determined the number and characteristics of the underlying dimensions. The scale developer, however, can use MDS as a first step, to reveal the 'psychological dimensions' people use in evaluating different stimuli, which are then used to construct scales that measure the various dimensions separately.

References

Aitken, R. C. B. (1969). A growing edge of measurement of feelings. *Proceedings of the Royal Society of Medicine*, **62**, 989–92.

Bosi Ferraz, M., Quaresma, M. R., Aquino, L. R. L., Atra, E., Tugwell, P., and Goldsmith, C. H. (1990). Reliability of pain scales in the assessment of literate and illiterate patients with rheumatoid arthritis. *Journal of Rheumatology*, **17**, 1022–4.

Bryant, G. D. and Norman, G. R. (1980). Expressions of probability: Words and numbers. *New England Journal of Medicine*, **302**, 411.

Dixon, P. N., Bobo, M., and Stevick, R. A. (1984). Response differences and preferences for all-category-defined and end-defined Likert formats. *Educational and Psychological Measurement*, **44**, 61–6.

Downie, W. W., Leatham, P. A., Rhind, V. M., Wright, V., Branco, J. A., and Anderson, J. A. (1978). Studies with pain rating scales. *Annals of Rheumatic Diseases*, **37**, 378–81.

Frisbie, D. A. and Brandenburg, D. C. (1979). Equivalence of questionnaire items with varying response formats. *Journal of Educational Measurement*, **16**, 43–8.

Gaito, J. (1982). Measurement scales and statistics: Resurgence of an old misconception. *Psychological Bulletin*, **87**, 564–7.

Guilford, J. P. (1954). *Psychometric methods*. McGraw-Hill, New York.

Harden, R. M. and Gleeson, F. A. (1979). Assessment of clinical experience using an objective structured clinical examination (OSCE). *Medical Education*, **13**, 41–54.

Hunter, J. E. and Schmidt, F. L. (1990). Dichotomization of continuous variables: The implications for meta-analysis. *Journal of Applied Psychology*, **75**, 334–49.

Huskisson, E. C. (1974). Measurement of pain. *Lancet*, **ii**, 1127–31.

Kiresuk, T. J. and Sherman, R. E. (1968). Goal attainment scaling: A general method for evaluating comprehensive community health programs. *Community Mental Health Journal*, **4**, 443–53.

Kruskal, J. B. and Wish, M. (1978). *Multidimensional scaling.* Sage, Beverly Hills, CA.

Lichtenstein, S. and Newman, J. R. (1967). Empirical scaling of common verbal phrases associated with numerical probabilities. *Psychonomic Science*, **9**, 563–4.

Likert, R. A. (1952). A technique for the development of attitude scales. *Educational and Psychological Measurement*, **12**, 313–15.

Llewellyn-Thomas, H. and Sutherland, H. (1986). Procedures for value assessment. In *Recent advances in nursing: Research methodology.* (ed. M. Calhoun) Churchill-Livingstone, London.

Miller, G. A. (1956). The magic number seven plus or minus two: Some limits on our capacity for processing information. *Psychological Bulletin*, **63**, 81–97.

Mohide, E. A., Torrance, G. W., Streiner, D. L., Pringle, D. M., and Gilbert, J. R. (1988). Measuring the well-being of family caregivers using the time tradeoff technique. *Journal of Clinical Epidemiology*, **41**, 475–82.

Newstead, S. E. and Arnold, J. (1989). The effect of response format on ratings of teachers. *Educational and Psychological Measurement*, **49**, 33–43.

Nishisato, N. and Torii, Y. (1970). Effects of categorizing continuous normal distributions on the product-moment correlation. *Japanese Psychological Research*, **13**, 45–9.

Norman, G. R. and Streiner, D. L. (1994). *Biostatistics: The bare essentials.* Mosby, St Louis, MO.

Osgood, C., Suci, G., and Tannenbaum, P. (1957). *The measurement of feeling.* University of Illinois Press, Urbana.

Santa-Barbara, J., Woodward, C. A., Levin, S., Goodman, J. T., Streiner, D. L., Muzzin, L. *et al.* (1974). Variables related to outcome in family therapy: Some preliminary analyses. *Goal Attainment Review*, **1**, 5–12.

Schaeffer, N. C. (1991). Hardly ever or constantly? Group comparisons using vague quantifiers. *Public Opinion Quarterly*, **55**, 395–423.

Schwarz, N., Knäuper, B., Hippler, H-J., Noelle-Neumann, E., and Clark, L. (1991). Rating scales: Numeric values may change the meaning of scale labels. *Public Opinion Quarterly*, **55**, 570–82.

Scott, P. J. and Huskisson, E. C. (1978). Measurement of functional capacity with visual analogue scales. *Rheumatology and Rehabilitation*, **16**, 257–9.

Scott, P. J. and Huskisson, E. C. (1979). Accuracy of subjective measurements made with and without previous scores: An important source of error in serial measurement of subjective states. *Annals of the Rheumatic Diseases*, **38**, 558–9.

Shearman, J. K., Evans, C. E. E., Boyle, M. H., Cuddy, L. J., and Norman, G. R. (1983). Maternal and infant characteristics in abuse: A case control study. *Journal of Family Practice*, **16**, 289–93.

Spector, P. E. (1976). Choosing response categories for summated rating scales. *Journal of Applied Psychology*, **61**, 374–5.

Stolee, P., Rockwood, K., Fox, R. A., and Streiner, D. L. (1992). The use of goal attainment scaling in a geriatric care setting. *Journal of the American Geriatric Society*, **40**, 574–8.

Suissa, S. (1991). Binary methods for continuous outcomes: A parametric alternative. *Journal of Clinical Epidemiology*, **44**, 241–8.

Torrance, G. (1976). Social preferences for health states: An empirical evaluation of three measurement techniques. *Socio-Economic Planning Sciences*, **10**, 129–36.

Torrance, G., Thomas, W. H., and Sackett, D. L. (1972). A utility maximization model for evaluation of health care programs. *Health Services Research*, **7**, 118–33.

Townsend, J. T. and Ashby, F. G. (1984). Measurement scales and statistics: The misconception misconceived. *Psychological Bulletin*, **96**, 394–401.

van der Vleuten, C. P., Norman, G. R., and de Graaff, E. (1991). Pitfalls in the pursuit of objectivity: Issues of reliability. *Medical Education*, **25**, 110–18.

Von Neumann, J. and Morgenstern, O. (1953). *The theory of games and economic behavior*. Wiley, New York.

Weinberg, S. L. (1991). An introduction to multidimensional scaling. *Measurement and Evaluation in Counseling and Development*, **24**, 12–36.

Wildt, A. R. and Mazis, A. B. (1978). Determinants of scale response: Label versus position. *Journal of Marketing Research*, **15**, 261–7.

5

Selecting the items

In previous chapters, we have discussed how to develop items which would be included in the new scale. Obviously, not all of the items will work as intended; some may be confusing to the respondent, some may not tell us what we thought they would, and so on. Here we examine various criteria used in determining which ones to retain and which to discard.

Interpretability

The first criterion for selecting items is to eliminate any which are ambiguous or incomprehensible. Problems can arise from any one of a number of sources: the words are too difficult; they contain jargon terms which are used only by certain groups of people, such as health professionals; or they are 'double-barrelled'.

Reading level

Except for scales which are aimed at a selected group whose educational level is known, the usual rule of thumb is that the scale should not require reading skills beyond that of a 12 year old. This may seem unduly low, but many people who are high-school graduates are unable to comprehend material much above this level. Many ways have been proposed to assess the reading level required to understand written material. Some methods, like the 'cloze' technique (Taylor 1957), eliminate every nth word to see at what point meaning disappears; the easier the material, the more words can be removed and accurately 'filled in' by the reader. Other methods are based on the number of syllables in each word or the number of words in each sentence (e.g. Flesch 1948; Fry 1968). However, these procedures can be laborious and time-consuming, and others may require up to 300 words of text (e.g. McLaughlin 1969). These are usually inappropriate for scales or questionnaires, where each item is an independent passage, and meaning may depend on one key word.

Within recent years, a number of computer packages have appeared which purport to check the grammar and style of one's writing. Some of these programs further provide one or more indices of reading level, and these have also been incorporated into various word processing packages. Since the procedures used in the programs are based on the techniques we just mentioned, their results should probably be interpreted with great caution when used to evaluate scales.

Another method is to use a list of words which are comprehensible at each grade level (e.g. Dale and Eichholz 1960). While it may be impractical (and even unnecessary) to check every word in the scale, those which appear to be difficult can be checked. Even glancing through one of these books can give the scale developer a rough idea of the complexity of Grade 6 words. Approaching the problem from the other direction, Payne (1954) compiled a very useful list of 1000 common words, indicating whether each was unambiguous, problematic, or had multiple meanings.

Ambiguity

This same method is often used to determine if the items are ambiguous or poorly worded. Even a seemingly straightforward item such as 'I like my mother', can pose a problem if the respondent's mother is dead. Some people answer by assuming that the sentence can also be read in the past tense, while others may simply say 'no', reflecting the fact that they can't like her now. On a questionnaire designed to assess patients' attitudes to their recent hospitalization, one item asked about information given to the patient by various people. A stem read 'I understand what was told to me by:', followed by a list of different health care professionals, with room to check either 'yes' or 'no'. Here, a 'no' response opposite 'Social Worker', for instance, could indicate

- that the patient did not understand what the social worker said,
- that she never saw a social worker, or
- that she does not remember whether she saw the social worker or not.

While these latter two possibilities were not what the test developer intended, the ambiguity of the question and the response scheme forced the subject to respond with an ambiguous answer.

Ambiguity can also arise by the vagueness of the response alternatives. The answer to the question, 'Have you seen your doctor recently' depends on the subject's interpretation of 'recently'. One person may feel that it refers to the previous week, another to the past month, and a third person may believe it covers the previous year. Even if we rephrase the question to use a seemingly more specific term, ambiguity can remain. 'Have you seen your doctor during the past year?' can mean

- during the last 12 months, more or less,
- since this date one year ago, or
- since 1 January of this year.

If a specific time frame (or any other variable) is called for, it should be spelled out explicitly. Questionnaire developers vastly overestimate people's ability to recall past events. The evidence is that people have difficulty remembering episodes of illness. Surprising as it may seem, the results of a major study showed that 42 per cent of people did not recall that they had been in hospital one year after the fact (United States National Health Survey 1965). In another study, there was a 22 per cent false positive rate and a 69 per cent false negative rate in the recall of serious medical events after one year, and a 32 per cent false positive and 53 per cent false negative rate for minor events (Means *et al.* 1989). The problem is even more severe if the people did not receive medical help for their illness (Allen *et al.* 1954). Drawing on cognitive theory (e.g. Neisser 1986; Linton 1975), Means *et al.* (1989) hypothesize that, especially for chronic conditions which result in recurring events, people have a 'generic memory' for the group of events and medical contacts, and therefore have difficulty recalling specific instances. Thus, the replies to questions like, 'Compared to how you felt a year ago . . . ' should be viewed with some degree of scepticism.

Double-barrelled question

A 'double-barrelled' item is one that asks two or more questions at the same time, each of which can be answered differently. These are unfortunately quite common in questionnaires probing for physical or psychological symptoms, such as 'My eyes are red and teary'. How should one answer if one's eyes are red but not teary or teary but not red? Since some people will say 'yes' only if both parts are true, while others will respond this way if either symptom was present, the final result may not reflect the actual state of affairs. Pre-testing on a large group, where it is likely that some people will fall into these grey areas, can reduce the risk of these types of items occurring.

Jargon

Jargon terms can slip into a scale or questionnaire quite insidiously. Since we use a technical vocabulary on a daily basis, and these terms are fully understood by our colleagues, it is easy to overlook the fact that these words are not part of the everyday vocabulary of others, or may have very different connotations. Terms like 'lesion', 'care-giver', or 'range of motion' may not be ones which the average person understands. Even more troublesome are words which *are* understood, but in a manner different from what the scale developer intended. 'Hypertension', for example, means 'being very tense' to some people; and asking some what colour their stool is may elicit the response that the problem is with their gut, not their furniture. Samora *et al.* (1961) compiled a list of 50 words which physicians said they used routinely with their patients, and then asked 125 patients to define them. Words which were erroneously defined at least 50 per cent of the time included 'nutrition', 'digestion', 'orally', and 'tissue'; words that most clinicians would assume their patients knew. The range of definitions given for *appendectomy* included a cut rectum, sickness, the stomach, a pain or disease, taking off an arm or leg, something contagious, or something to do with the bowels, in addition to surgical removal of the appendix. Patients and physicians differ even in terms of what should be called a disease. Campbell *et al.*

(1979) state that 'the medically qualified were consistently more generous in their acceptance of disease connotation than the laymen' (p. 760). Over 90 per cent of general practitioners, for instance, called duodenal ulcers a disease, while only 50 per cent of lay people did. Boyle (1970) found the greatest disagreement between physicians and patients to be in the area of the location of internal organs. Nearly 58 per cent of patients had the heart occupying the entire thorax, or being adjacent to the left shoulder (almost 2 per cent had it near the right shoulder). Similarly, the majority of patients placed the stomach over the belly button, somewhat south of its actual location. Not surprisingly, knowledge of medical terms, and the aetiology, treatment, and symptoms of various disorders, is strongly associated with educational level (Seligman *et al.* 1957). Again, pre-testing is desirable, with the interviewer asking the people not whether they had the complaint, but rather what they think the term means.

Value-laden words

A final factor affecting the interpretation of the question is the use of value-laden terms. Items such as 'Do you often go to your doctor with trivial problems?' or 'Do physicians make too much money?' may prejudice the respondents, leading them to answer as much to the tenor of the question as to its content. (Both items also contain ambiguous terms, such as 'often', 'trivial', and 'too much'.) Naturally, such value-laden terms should be avoided.

Positive and negative wording

As a general rule, scale developers should avoid negatively worded items; that is, items which use words such as 'not', 'rarely', or 'never', or which have words with negative prefixes (e.g., in-, im-, or un-). Such items tend to have lower validity coefficients than positively worded ones (Holden *et al.* 1985; Schriesheim and Hill 1981). It would be better to have an item which states 'I feel ill most of the time', for example, rather than 'I rarely feel well'.

Length of items

Items on scales should be as short as possible, although not so short that comprehensibility is lost. Item validity coefficients tend to fall as the number of letters in the item increases. Holden *et al.* (1985) found that, on average, items with 70–80 letters had validity coefficients under 0.10, while items containing 10–20 characters had coefficients almost four times higher.

Testing the questions

Having obeyed all of these rules, there is still no guarantee that the questions will be interpreted by the subjects as they were intended to be. Belson (1981), for example, found that fewer than 30 per cent of survey questions were correctly interpreted by readers. Unfortunately, these results are typical of findings in this area.

Perhaps the best way to ensure that the items are understood, unambiguous, and jargon-free is to pretest them on a group of people comparable to those who will be the ultimate targets. Following a technique introduced by Nuckols (1953), the people are asked to rephrase the question in their own words, trying to keep the meaning as close to the original as possible. The responses, which are written down verbatim, are later coded into one of four categories: fully correct; generally correct (no more than one part altered or omitted); partially wrong (but the person understood the intent); and completely wrong (Foddy 1993). Other techniques which can be used to test the subjects' understanding of the items are the *double interview* and *asking people to think aloud*. In the first method, the entire questionnaire is given. Then, for each subject, three or four questions are selected, and the interviewer asks questions such as, 'What led you to answer . . . ' or 'Tell me exactly how you came to that answer' (Foddy 1993). In the second technique, the subjects are asked to think aloud as they formulate their responses. Naturally, all of these approaches can be used for the same items, with different groups of respondents.

In all cases, though, it is important that the subjects are representative of the people who will ultimately be completing the questionnaire. Using one's colleagues or samples of convenience, which may bear little resemblance to the final user population, will most likely result in underestimating any potential problems.

Rechecking

Even after all of the items have passed these checks and have been incorporated into the scale, it is worthwhile to check them over informally every year or so to see if any terms may have taken on new meanings. For example, liking to go to 'gay parties' has a very different connotation now than it did some years ago, when to most people the word 'gay' had no association with homosexuality.

Face validity

One issue that must be decided before the items are written or selected is whether or not they should have *face validity*. That is, do the items appear on the surface to be measuring what they actually are? As is often the case, there are two schools of thought on this issue, and the 'correct' answer often depends on the purpose that the measure will be used for.

Those who argue for face validity state, quite convincingly, that it increases the acceptance of the instrument by those who will ultimately use it. If the item appears irrelevant, then the respondent may very well object to it or omit it, irrespective of its possibly superb psychometric properties. For example, it is commonly believed that some psychiatric patients manifest increased religiosity, especially during the acute phase of their illness. Capitalizing on this fact, the MMPI contains a few items tapping into this domain. Despite the fact that these items are psychometrically quite good, it has opened the test to much (perhaps unnecessary) criticism for delving into seemingly irrelevant, private matters.

On the other hand, it may be necessary in some circumstances to disguise the true nature of the question, lest the respondents try to 'fake' their answers, an issue we will return to in greater detail in Chapter 6. For example, patients may want to appear worse than they actually are in order to ensure that they will receive help; or better than they really feel in order to please the doctor. This is easy to do if the items have face validity—that is, their meaning and relevance are self-evident—and much harder if they do not. Thus, the ultimate decision depends on the nature and purpose of the instrument.

Frequency of endorsement and discrimination

After the scale has been pretested for readability and absence of ambiguity, it is then given to a large group of subjects to test for other attributes, including the endorsement frequency. (The meaning of 'large' is variable, but usually 50 subjects would be an absolute minimum.) The frequency of endorsement is simply the proportion of people (p) who give each response alternative to an item. For dichotomous items, this reduces to simply the proportion saying 'yes' (or, conversely, 'no'). A multiple-choice item has a number of 'frequencies of endorsement;' the proportion choosing alternative A, one for alternative B, and so forth.

In achievement tests, the frequency of endorsement is a function of the *difficulty* of the item, with a specific response alternative reflecting the correct answer. For personality measures, the frequency of endorsement is the 'popularity' of that item; the proportion of people who choose the alternative which indicates more of the trait, attitude, or behaviour (Allen and Yen 1979).

Usually, items where one alternative has a very high (or low) endorsement rates are eliminated. If p is over 0.95 (or under 0.05), then most people are responding in the same direction or with the same alternative. Since we can predict what the answer will be with greater than 95 per cent accuracy, we learn very little by knowing how a person actually responded. Such questions do not improve a scale's psychometric properties, and may actually detract from them while making the test longer. In practice, only items with endorsement rates between 0.20 and 0.80 are used.

There are some scales, though, which are deliberately made up of items with a high endorsement frequency. This is the case where there may be some question regarding the subject's ability or willingness to answer honestly. A person may not read the item accurately because of factors such as illiteracy, retardation, or difficulties in concentration; or may not answer honestly because of an attempt to 'fake' a response for some reason. Some tests, like the MMPI or the *Personality Research Form* (Jackson 1984), have special scales to detect these biases, comprised of a heterogeneous group of items which have only one thing in common: an endorsement frequency of 90–95 per cent. To get rates this high, the questions have to be either quite bizarre (e.g. 'I have never touched money') or extremely banal ('I eat most days'). A significant number of questions answered in the 'wrong' direction is a flag that the person was not reading the items carefully and responding as would most people. This may temper the interpretation given to other scales that the person completes.

Another index of the utility of an item, closely related to endorsement frequency, is its *discrimination* ability. This tells us if a person who has a high total score is more likely to have endorsed the item; conversely, if the item discriminates between those who score high (and supposedly have more of the trait) and those who score low. It is related to endorsement frequency in that, from a psychometric viewpoint, items which discriminate best among people have values of p near the cut-point of the scale. It differs in that it looks at the item in relation to all of the other items on the scale, not just in isolation.

A simple item discrimination index is given by the formula

$$d_i = \frac{U_i - L_i}{n_i},$$

where U_i is the number of people above the median who score positive on item i, L_i is the number of people below the median who score positive on item i, and n_i is the number of people above (or below) the median.

Homogeneity of the items

In most situations, whenever we are measuring a trait, behaviour, or symptom, we want the scale to be homogeneous. That is, all of the items should be tapping different aspects of the same attribute, and not different parts of different traits. (Later in this chapter we deal with the situation where we want the test to measure a variety of characteristics.) For example, if we were measuring the problem-solving ability of medical students, then each item should relate to problem solving. This has two implications:
- the items should be moderately correlated with each other, and
- each should correlate with the total scale score.

Indeed, these two factors form the basis of the various tests of homogeneity or 'internal consistency' of the scale.

Before the mechanics of measuring internal consistency are discussed, some rationale and background are in order. In almost all areas we measure, a simple summing of the scores over the individual items is the most sensible index; this point will be returned to in Chapter 7. However, this 'linear model' approach (Nunnally 1970) works only if all items are measuring the same trait. If the items were measuring different attributes, it would not be logical to add them up to form one total score. On the other hand, if one item were highly correlated with a second one, then the latter question would add little additional information. Hence there is a need to derive some quantitative measure of the degree to which items are related to each other; i.e. the degree of 'homogeneity' of the scale.

Current thinking in test development holds that there should be a moderate correlation among the items in a scale. If the items were chosen without regard for homogeneity, then the resulting scale could possibly end up tapping a number of traits. If the correlations were too high, there would be much redundancy, and a possible loss of content validity.

It should be noted that this position of taking homogeneity into account, which is most closely identified with Jackson (1970) and Nunnally (1970), is not shared by all psychometricians. Another school of thought is that internal consistency and face validity make sense if the primary aim is to *describe* a trait, behaviour, or disorder, but not necessarily if the goal is to *discriminate* people who have an attribute from those who do not. That is, if we are trying to measure the degree of depression, for example, the scale should *appear* to be measuring it and all of the items should relate to this in a coherent manner. On the other hand, if our aim is to *discriminate* depressed patients from other groups, then it is sufficient to choose items which are answered differently by the depressed group, irrespective of their content. This in fact was the method used in constructing the MMPI, one of the most famous paper-and-pencil questionnaires for psychological assessment. An item was included in the Depression Scale (*D*) based on the criterion that depressed patients responded to it in one way significantly more often than did non-depressed people, and without regard for the correlation among the individual items. As a result, the *D* scale has some items which seem to be related to depression, but also many other items which do not. On the other hand, the more recent CES-D (Radloff 1977), which measures depressive symptomatology without diagnosing depression, was constructed following the philosophy of high internal consistency, and its items all appear to be tapping into this domain. If a trend can be detected, it is toward scales that are more grounded in theory and are more internally consistent, and away from the empiricism that led to the MMPI.

One last comment is in order before discussing the techniques of item selection. Many inventories, especially those in the realms of psychology and psychiatry, are multidimensional; that is, they are comprised of a number of different scales, with the items intermixed in a random manner. Measures of homogeneity should be applied to the individual scales, as it does not make sense to talk of homogeneity across different subscales.

Item–total correlation

One of the oldest, albeit still widely used, methods for checking the homogeneity of the scale is the *item–total correlation*. As the name implies, it is the correlation of the individual item with the scale total *omitting that item*. If we did not remove the item from the total score, the correlation would be artificially inflated, since it would be based in part on the item correlated with itself. The item can be eliminated in one of two ways; physically or statistically. We can physically remove the item by not including it when calculating the total score. So, for a five-item scale, Item 1 would be correlated with the sum of Items 2–5; Item 2 with the sum of 1 and 3–5; and so on. One problem with this approach is that, for a *k*-item scale, we have to calculate the total score *k* times; not a difficult problem, but a laborious one, especially if a computer program to do this is not readily available.

The second method is statistical; the item's contribution to the total score is removed using the formula given by Nunnally (1978):

$$r_{i(t-1)} = \frac{r_{it}\,\sigma_t - \sigma_i}{\sqrt{(\sigma_i^2 + \sigma_t^2 - 2\sigma_i\,\sigma_t\,r_{it})}},$$

where $r_{i(t-1)}$ is the correlation of item i with the total, removing the effect of item i, r_{it} is the correlation of item i with the total score, σ_i is the standard deviation of item i; and σ_t is the standard deviation of the total score.

The usual rule of thumb is that an item should correlate with the total score above 0.20. Items with lower correlations should be discarded (Kline 1986).

In almost all instances, the best coefficient to use is the *Pearson product-moment correlation* (Nunnally 1970). If the items are dichotomous, then the usually recommended point-biserial correlation yields identical results; if there are more than two response alternatives, the product-moment correlation is robust enough to produce relatively accurate results, even if the data are not normally distributed (see for example Havlicek and Peterson 1977).

Split-half reliability

Another approach to testing the homogeneity of a scale is called *split-half reliability*. Here, the items are randomly divided into two sub-scales, which are then correlated with each other. This is also referred to as 'odd—even' reliability, since the easiest split is to put all odd-numbered items in one half and even-numbered ones in the other. If the scale is internally consistent, then the two halves should correlate highly.

One problem is that the resulting correlation is an underestimate of the true reliability of the scale, since the reliability of a scale is directly proportional to the number of items in it. Since the sub-scales being correlated are only half the length of the version that will be used in practice, the resulting correlation will be too low. The Spearman–Brown 'prophesy' formula is used to correct for this occurrence. The equation for this is

$$r_{SB} = \frac{kr}{1 + (k-1)r},$$

where k is the factor by which the scale is to be increased or decreased, and r is the original correlation.

In this case, we want to see the result when there are twice the number of items, so k is set at 2. For example, if we found that splitting a 40-item scale in half yields a correlation of 0.50, we would substitute into the equation as follows:

$$r_{SB} = \frac{2 \times 0.50}{1 + (2-1) \times 0.50}.$$

Thus, the estimate of the split-half reliability of this scale would be 0.67.

Since there are many ways to divide a test into two parts, there are in fact many possible split-half reliabilities; a 10-item test can be divided 126 ways, a 12-item test 462 different ways, and so on. (These numbers represent the combination of n items taken $n/2$ at a time. This is then divided by 2, since (assuming a six-item scale) items 1, 2, and 3 in the first half and 4, 5, and 6 in the second is the same as 4, 5, and 6 in the first part and the remaining items in the second.) These reliability coefficients may differ quite considerably from one split to another.

There are two situations where we should *not* divide a test randomly; highly timed achievement tests, and tests with serially related items. In the former case, where the major emphasis is on how quickly a person can work, most of the items are fairly easy, and failure is due to not reaching that question before the time limit. Thus, the answers up to the timed cut-off will almost all be correct, and those after it all incorrect. Any split-half reliability will yield a very high value, only marginally lower than 1.0.

With related or 'chained' items, failure on the second item could occur in two ways: not being able to answer it correctly; or being able to do it, but getting it wrong, because of an erroneous response to the previous item. For example, assume that the two (relatively simple) items were:

A. The organ for pumping blood is:
  1. The pineal gland
  2. The heart
  3. The stomach

B. It is located in:
  1. The chest
  2. The gut
  3. The skull

If the answer to A were correct, then a wrong response to B would indicate that the person did not know where the heart is located. However, if A and B were wrong, then the person *may* have known that the heart is located in the chest, but went astray in believing that blood is pumped by the pineal gland. Whenever this can occur, it is best to keep both items in the same half of the scale.

Kuder-Richardson 20 and Coefficient α

There are two problems in using split-half reliability to determine which items to retain. First, as we have just seen, there are many ways to divide a test; and second, it does not tell us which item(s) may be contributing to a low reliability. Both of these problems are addressed with two related techniques, *Kuder-Richardson formula 20* (KR-20; Kuder and Richardson 1937) and *Coefficient α* (also called Cronbach's alpha; Cronbach 1951).

KR-20 is appropriate for scales with items which are answered dichotomously, such as 'true—false', 'yes—no', 'present—absent', and so forth. To compute it, the proportion of people answering positively to each of the questions and the standard deviation of the total score must be known, and then put into the formula

$$\text{KR-20} = \frac{n}{n-1}\left(1 - \frac{\Sigma\, p_i q_i}{\sigma_T^2}\right),$$

where n is the number of items, p_i is the proportion answering correctly to question i, $q_i = (1 - p)$ for each item, and σ_T is the standard deviation of the total score.

Cronbach's α (alpha) is an extension of KR-20, allowing it to be used when there are more than two response alternatives. If α were used with dichotomous items, the result would be identical to that obtained with KR-20. The formula for α is very similar to KR-20, except that the standard deviation for each item (σ_i) is substituted for $p_i q_i$:

$$\alpha = \frac{n}{n-1}\left(1 - \frac{\Sigma\, \sigma_i^2}{\sigma_T^2}\right).$$

Conceptually, both equations give the average of all of the possible split-half reliabilities of a scale. Their advantage in terms of scale development is that, especially with the use of computers, it is possible to do them n times, each time omitting one item. If KR-20 or α increases significantly when a specific item is left out, this would indicate that its exclusion would increase the homogeneity of the scale.

It is nearly impossible these days to see a scale development paper that has not used α, and the implication is usually made that the higher the coefficient, the better. However, there are problems in uncritically accepting high values of α (or KR-20), and especially in interpreting them as reflecting simply internal consistency. The first problem is that α is dependent not only on the magnitude of the correlations among the items, but also on the number of items in the scale. A scale can be made to look more 'homogeneous' simply by doubling the number of items, even though the average correlation remains the same. This leads directly to the second problem. If we have two scales which each measure a distinct construct, and combine them to form one long scale, α would probably be high, although the merged scale is obviously tapping two different attributes. Third, if α is too high, then it may suggest a high level of item redundancy; that is, a number of items asking the same question in slightly different ways (Boyle 1991; Hattie 1985). This may indicate that some of the items are unnecessary, and that the scale as a whole may be too narrow in its scope to have much validity. Thus, α should be above 0.70 (Nunnally 1978), but probably not higher than 0.90.

Multifactor inventories

If the scale is one part of an inventory which has a number of other scales (usually called 'multifactor' or 'multidimensional' inventories), more sophisticated item analytic techniques are possible. The first is an extension of the item—total procedure, in which the item is correlated with its scale total, *and with the totals of all of the other scales*. The item should meet the criteria outlined above for a single index; additionally, this correlation should be higher than with any of the scales it is *not* included in.

The second technique is *factor analysis*. Very briefly, this statistic is predicated on the belief that a battery of tests can be described in terms of a smaller number of underlying factors. For example, assume students were given five tests: vocabulary, word fluency, verbal analogies, mechanical reasoning, and arithmetic. It might be expected that their scores on the first three tasks would be correlated with one another, that the last two would be correlated, but that the two sets of scores would not necessarily be related to each other. That is, high scores on the first three may or may not be associated with high scores on the latter two. We would postulate that the first group reflected a 'verbal' factor, and the second a 'reasoning' one. (For more details presented in a non-mathematical fashion, see Norman and Streiner 1986; for even more detail, see Harman 1976).

In an analogous manner, each item in a multifactorial test could be treated as an individual 'test'. Ideally, then, there should be as many factors as separate scales in the inventory. The item should 'load on' (i.e. be correlated with) the scale it belongs to, and not on any other one. If it loads on the 'wrong' factor, or on two or more factors, then it is likely that it may be tapping something other than what the developer intended, and should be either rewritten or discarded.

More recent developments in factor analysis allow the test developer to specify beforehand what he or she thinks the final structure of the test should look like. The results show how closely the observed pattern corresponds to this hypothesized pattern (Darton 1980). Although factor analysis has been used quite often with dichotomous items, this practice is highly suspect, and can lead to quite anomalous results (Comrey 1978).

Putting it all together

In outline form, these are the steps involved in the initial selection of items:

A. Pre-test the items to ensure that they:
  1. are comprehensible to the target population,
  2. are unambiguous, and
  3. ask only a single question.

B. Eliminate or rewrite any items which do not meet these criteria, and pretest again.

C. Discard items endorsed by very few (or very many) subjects.

D. Check for the internal consistency of the scale using:
  1. Item–Total correlation
     (a) Correlate each item with the scale total omitting that item.
     (b) Eliminate or rewrite any with Pearson r's less than 0.20.
     (c) Rank order the remaining ones and select items starting with the highest correlation.

or

  2. Coefficient α or KR-20
     (a) Calculate α eliminating one item at a time.
     (b) Discard any item where α significantly increases.

E. For multiscale questionnaires, check that the item is in the 'right' scale by:
  1. Correlating it with the totals of all the scales, eliminating items which correlate more highly on scales other than the one it belongs to; or
  2. Factor-analysing the questionnaire, eliminating items which load more highly on other factors than the one it should belong to.

References

Allen, G. I., Breslow, L., Weissman, A., and Nisselson, H. (1954). Interviewing versus diary keeping in eliciting information in a morbidity survey. *American Journal of Public Health*, **44**, 919–27.

Allen, M. J. and Yen, W. M. (1979). *Introduction to measurement theory*. Brooks/Cole, Monterey, CA.

Belson, W. A. (1981). *The design and understanding of survey questions*. Gower, Aldershot.

Boyle, C. M. (1970). Differences between patients' and doctors' interpretation of some common medical terms. *British Medical Journal*, **2**, 286–9.

Boyle, G. J. (1991). Does item homogeneity indicate internal consistency or item redundancy in psychometric scales? *Personality and Individual Differences*, **12**, 291–4.

Campbell, E. J. M., Scadding, J. G., and Roberts, R. S. (1979). The concept of disease. *British Medical Journal*, **ii**, 757–62.

Comrey, A. L. (1978). Common methodological problems in factor analysis. *Journal of Consulting and Clinical Psychology*, **46**, 648–59.

Cronbach, L. J. (1951). Coefficient alpha and the internal structure of tests. *Psychometrika*, **16**, 297–334.

Dale, E. and Eichholz, G. (1960). *Children's knowledge of words*. Ohio State University, Columbus, OH.

Darton, R. A. (1980). Rotation in factor analysis. *The Statistician*, **29**, 167–94.

Flesch, R. (1948). A new readability yardstick. *Journal of Applied Psychology*, **32**, 221–33.

Foddy, W. (1993). *Constructing questions for interviews and questionnaires*. Cambridge University Press, Cambridge.

Fry, E. A. (1968). A readability formula that saves time. *Journal of Reading*, **11**, 513–16.

Harman, H. H. (1976). *Modern factor analysis* (3rd edn). University of Chicago Press, Chicago.

Hattie, J. (1985). Methodology review: Assessing unidimensionality of tests and items. *Applied Psychological Measurement*, **9**, 139–64.

Havlicek, L. L. and Peterson, N. L. (1977). Effect of the violation of assumptions upon significance levels of the Pearson *r*. *Psychological Bulletin*, **84**, 373–77.

Holden, R. R., Fekken, G. C., and Jackson, D. N. (1985). Structured personality test item characteristics and validity. *Journal of Research in Personality*, **19**, 386–94.

Jackson, D. N. (1970). A sequential system for personality scale development. In *Current topics in clinical and community psychology*, (ed. C. D. Spielberger) Vol. 2, pp. 61–96. Academic Press, New York.

Jackson, D. N. (1984). *Personality Research Form manual*. Research Psychologists Press, Port Huron MI.

Kline, P. (1986). *A handbook of test construction*. Methuen, London.

Kuder, G. F. and Richardson, M. W. (1937). The theory of estimation of test reliability. *Psychometrika*, **2**, 151–60.

Linton, M. (1975). Memory for real world events. In *Explorations in cognition* (eds. D. A. Norman and D. E. Rumelhart) pp. 376–404. Freeman, San Francisco.

McLaughlin, G. H. (1969). SMOG grading: A new readability formula. *Journal of Reading*, **12**, 639–46.

Means, B., Nigam, A., Zarrow, M., Loftus, E. F., and Donaldson, M. S. (1989). Autobiographical memory for health-related events. *Vital and health statistics*, Series 6: Cognition and Survey Measurement, No. 2. Public Health Service, Hyattsville, MD.

Neisser, U. (1986). Nested structure in autobiographical memory. In *Autobiographical memory* (ed. D. C. Rubin) pp. 71–81. Cambridge University Press, Cambridge.

Norman, G. R. and Streiner, D. L. (1986). *PDQ statistics*. B. C. Decker, Toronto.

Nuckols, R. C. (1953). A note on pre-testing public opinion questions. *Journal of Applied Psychology*, **37**, 119–20.

Nunnally, J. C., Jr. (1970). *Introduction to psychological measurement*. McGraw-Hill, New York.

Nunnally, J. C., Jr. (1978). *Psychometric theory* (2nd edn). McGraw-Hill, New York.

Payne, S. L. (1954) *The art of asking questions*. Princeton University Press, Princeton NJ.

Radloff, L. S. (1977). The CES-D scale: A self-report depression scale for research in the general population. *Applied Psychological Measurement*, **1**, 385–401.

Samora, J., Saunders, L., and Larson, R. F. (1961). Medical vocabulary knowledge among hospital patients. *Journal of Health and Human Behavior*, **2**, 83–92.

Schriesheim, C. A. and Hill, K. D. (1981). Controlling acquiescence response bias by item reversals: The effect on questionnaire validity. *Educational and Psychological Measurement*, **41**, 1101–14.

Seligman, A. W., McGrath, N. E., and Pratt, L. (1957). Level of medical information among clinic patients. *Journal of Chronic Diseases*, **6**, 497–509.

Taylor, W. L. (1957). 'Cloze' readability scores as indices of individual differences in comprehension and aptitude. *Journal of Applied Psychology*, **41**, 19–26.

United States National Health Survey (1965). *Reporting of hospitalization in the Health Interview Survey*. Health Statistics, Series 3, No. 6. Public Health Service, Hyattsville, MD.

6

Biases in responding

When an item is included in a questionnaire or scale, it is usually under the assumption that the respondent will answer honestly. However, there has been considerable research, especially since the 1950s, showing that there are numerous factors which may influence a response, making it a less than totally accurate reflection of reality. The magnitude and seriousness of the problem depends very much on the nature of the instrument and the conditions under which it is used. At the extreme, questionnaires may end up over- or under-estimating the prevalence of a symptom or disease; or the validity of the scale may be seriously jeopardized.

Some scale developers bypass the entire problem of responder bias by asserting that their instruments are designed merely to differentiate between groups. In this situation, the truth or falsity of the answer is irrelevant, as long as one group responds in one direction more often than does another group. According to this position, responding 'yes' to an item such as 'I like sports magazines' would not be interpreted as accurately reflecting the person's reading preferences. The item's inclusion in the test is predicated solely on the fact that one group of people *says* it likes these magazines more often than do other groups. This purely empirical approach to scale development reached its zenith in the late 1940s and 1950s, but may still be found underlying the construction of some measures.

However, with the gradual trend toward instruments which are more grounded in theory, this approach to scale construction has become less appealing. The objective now is to reduce bias in responding as much as possible. In this chapter, we will examine some of the sources of error, what effects they may have on the scale, and how to minimize them.

The differing perspectives

The people who develop a scale, those who use it in their work, and the ones who are asked to fill it out, all approach scales from different perspectives, for different reasons, and with differing amounts of information about the instrument. For the person administering the instrument, a specific answer to a given question is often of little interest. That item may be just one of many on a scale, where the important information is the total score, and there is little regard for the individual items which have contributed to it. In other situations, the responses may be aggregated across dozens or hundreds of subjects, so that the individual person's answers are buried in a mass of those from other anonymous subjects. Further, what the questioner wants is 'truth'—did the person have this symptom or not, ever engage in this behaviour or not, and so forth. The clinician cannot help the patient, or the researcher discover important facts, unless honest answers are given. Moreover, the assessment session is perceived, at least in the assessors' minds, as non-judgmental and their attitude as disinterested. This may appear so obvious to scale developers that it never occurs to them that the respondents may perceive the situation from another angle.

The respondents' perspectives, however, are often quite different. They are often unaware that the individual items are ignored in favour of the total score. Even when told that their responses will be scored by a computer, it is quite common to find marginal notes explaining or elaborating their answers. Thus, it appears that respondents treat each item as important in its own right, and often believe that their answers will be read and evaluated by another person.

Additionally, their motivation may include the very natural tendency to be seen in a good light; or to be done with this intrusion in their lives as quickly as possible; or to ensure that they receive the help they feel they need. As we will discuss, these and other factors may influence the response given.

Optimizing and satisficing

Asking a seemingly simply question, such as 'How strongly do you feel that you should never spank a child?', requires the respondent to undertake a fairly complex cognitive task. According to some theories (e.g. Tourangeau 1984), there are at least four steps that people must go through. First, they must try to interpret the meaning of the question itself. Does 'spank' mean slapping the child's hand once if he puts it too near the stove, or is it limited to repeated hits on the backside which results in the child crying? Does the response option 'strongly agree' mean it should never be done at all, or that spanking can be used rarely and in extreme circumstances? And so on. The next step is that the respondents try to retrieve all relevant information from their memories. Did they ever spank their children? If so, how often did it occur and under what circumstances? How did they feel about it afterwards, and what were they told about spanking by their parents and spouse? Third, they must take the information they retrieved, which is often contradictory, and use it to form a single, integrated summary judgement. Last, they must try to convey that judgement on the answer sheet, which perhaps uses a format with which they are unfamiliar or uncomfortable. Borrowing a term from economic decision making (Simon 1957), Krosnick (1991) uses the term *optimizing* to describe the performance of these tasks in a careful and comprehensive manner.

The hope of the scale developer is that all of the respondents will use an optimizing strategy as they answer each of the items on the questionnaire. However, as we outlined in the previous section, the aims of the person who developed the scale and those of the person filling it out are not the same. Especially if the questionnaire is long, the items require considerable cognitive effort to answer them, and the purpose of filling it out is seemingly trivial or irrelevant to the respondents, they may adopt a strategy which allows them to complete the task without as much effort. Using another economic decision making term, Krosnick calls this *satisficing*; giving an answer which is satisfactory (that is, a box on the form is filled in), but not optimal. He describes six ways in which satisficing may occur. He refers to the first two as 'weak' forms, in that some cognitive effort is required; whereas the last four are 'strong' types of satisficing, since little or no thought is required.

First, the person may select the first response option that seems reasonable. If the options are presented in written form, the respondent will opt for the one that occurs first, and give only cursory attention to those which appear later. Conversely, if the options are given verbally, it is easier to remember those which came most recently; that is, those toward the end of the list. In either case, the choices in the middle get short shrift. Awareness of this phenomenon has led some organizations to minimize its effects in balloting. Recognizing that most voters do not know the people running for office, except for the long and often boring (and unread) position statements they write, and that the task of choosing among them is difficult and seemingly irrelevant for many voters, there is a danger that those whose names are closer to the top of the ballot will receive more votes. Consequently, organizations have adopted the strategy of using multiple forms of the ballot, with the names randomized differently on each version.

A second form of satisficing consists of simply agreeing with every statement, or answering 'true' or 'false' to each item. We will return to this bias later in this chapter, in the section on yea-saying and acquiescence.

Third, the person may endorse the status quo. This is not usually a problem when asking people about their physical or psychological state or about behaviours they may or may not do, but can be an issue when enquiring about their attitudes toward some policy. Having been asked their opinion about, for instance, whether certain procedures should be covered by universal health insurance or if we should allow *in vitro* fertilization of single women, it is easier to say 'keep things as they are' rather than considering the effects of change.

A fourth strategy is to select one answer for the first item, and then to use this response for all of the subsequent questions. This is a particular problem when the response options consist of visual analogue or Likert scales keyed in the same direction, so that the person simply has to go down the page in a straight line, putting check marks on each line. The trade-off is that changing the options for each question may minimize this tendency (or at least make it more obvious to the scorer), but it places an additional cognitive demand on the subject, which further fosters satisficing.

Fifth, the person may simply say 'I don't know' or place a mark in a neutral point along a Likert scale. In some circumstances, it may be possible to eliminate these alternatives, such as by using a scale with an even number of boxes, as we described in Chapter 4. However, these may be valid options for some optimizing subjects, and their removal may make their responses less valid.

The last way a person may satisfice is to mentally flip a coin; that is, to choose a response at random. Krosnick (1991) believes that this is the 'method of last resort', and used only when the previous ones cannot be.

There are two general ways to minimize satisficing. First, the task should be kept as simple as possible. At the most superficial level, this means that the questions should be kept short and the words easy to understand; points covered in Chapter 5. Further, the mental processes required to answer the question should not be overly demanding. For example, it is easier to say how you currently feel about something than how you felt about it in the past; less difficult to remember what you did for the past month than over the past year; and how you feel about one thing rather than comparing two or more, since each requires its own retrieval and evaluation process. Last, the response options should not be overly complex, but must include all possibilities. If there are even a few questions which do not have appropriate answers for some subjects, they may stop trying to give the optimal answer and start satisficing.

The second way to decrease satisficing is to maintain the motivation of the respondents. One way is to include only individuals who are interested in the topic, rather than using samples of convenience. Second, recognize that motivation is usually higher at the start of a task, and begins to flag as it gets longer and more onerous. Consequently, instruments should be kept as short as possible. (However, as we will see in Chapter 13, 'short' can be up to 100 items or 10 pages.) A third way is to make the respondents accountable for their answers; that is, they feel that they may have to justify what they said. This can be accomplished by asking them to explain why they gave the answer which they did. Last, motivation can be provided externally, by rewarding them for their participation; we will also discuss this further in Chapter 13.

Social desirability and faking good

A person's answer to an item like, 'During an average day, how much alcohol do you consume?' or 'I am a shy person' may not correspond to what an outside observer would say about that individual. In many cases, people give a socially desirable answer; the drinker may minimize his daily intake, or the retiring person may deny it, believing it is better to be outgoing. As *social desirability* is commonly conceptualized, the subject is not deliberately trying to deceive or lie; he or she is unaware of this tendency to put the best foot forward (Edwards 1957). When the person *is* aware and is intentionally attempting to create a false positive impression, it is called *faking good*. Although conceptually different, the two biases create similar problems for the scale developer, and have similar solutions.

Social desirability (SD) depends on many factors: the individual, the person's sex and cultural background, the specific question, and the context in which the item is asked; e.g. face-to-face interview versus an anonymous questionnaire. Sudman and Bradburn (1982) derived a list of threatening topics which are prone to SD bias. Among the 'socially desirable' ones apt to lead to over-reporting are being a good citizen (e.g. registering to vote and voting, knowing issues in public debates), being well-informed and cultured (e.g. reading news-papers and books, using the library, attending cultural activities), and having ful-filled moral and social responsibilities (e.g. giving to charity, helping friends and relatives). Conversely, there will be under-reporting of 'socially undesirable' topics, such as certain illnesses and disabilities (e.g. cancer, sexually transmitted diseases, mental disorders), illegal and non-normative behaviours (e.g. commit-ting a crime, tax evasion, use of drugs and alcohol, non-marital sex), and finan-cial status (income, savings, having expensive possessions).

A debate has raged for many years whether SD is a trait (whereby the person responds in the desirable direction irrespective of the context) or a state (depen-dent more on the question and the setting). While the jury is still out, two suggestions have emerged: SD should be minimized whenever possible, and the person's propensity to respond in this manner should be assessed whenever it may affect how he or she answers (e.g. Anastasi 1982; Jackson 1984).

If answers are affected by social desirability, the validity of the scale may be jeopardized for two reasons. First, if the object of the questionnaire is to gather factual information, such as the prevalence of a disorder, behaviour, or feeling, then the results obtained may not reflect the true state of affairs. The prime example of this would be items tapping socially sanctioned acts, like drug taking, premarital sexual relations, or abortions; but SD may also affect responses to embarrassing, unpopular, or 'unacceptable' feelings, such as anger towards one's parents, or admitting to voting for the party which lost the last election (or won, depending on recent events). In a similar fashion, the occurrence of posi-tive or socially desired behaviours may be overestimated.

The second problem, to which we will return in Chapter 10, involves what is called the 'discriminant validity' of a test. Very briefly, if a scale correlates highly with one factor (e.g. SD), then that limits how highly it can correlate with the factor which the scale was designed to assess. Further, the theoretical rationale of the scale is undermined, since the most parsimonious explanation of what the test is measuring would be 'social desirability', rather than anything else.

The social desirability of an item can be assessed in a number of ways. One method is to correlate each item on a new instrument with a scale specifically designed to measure this tendency. Jackson (1970) has developed an index called the *Differential Reliability Index* (DRI), defined as

$$\text{DRI} = \sqrt{(r_{is}^2 - r_{id}^2)},$$

where r_{is} is the item-scale correlation, and r_{id} is the item–SD correlation.

The DRI in essence is the difference between the item–total correlation and the item–SD correlation. Any item which is more highly 'saturated' on SD than with its scale total will result in a DRI approaching zero (note that if r_{id} is ever larger than r_{is}, DRI is undefined). Such an item should either be rewritten or discarded.

A number of scales have been developed to specifically measure the tendency to give socially desirable answers. These include the Crowne and Marlowe (1960) *Social Desirability Scale*, which is perhaps the most widely used such instrument; the *Desirability* (DY) scale on the *Personality Research Form* (Jackson 1984); and one developed by Edwards (1957). These are sometimes given in conjunction with other scales, not so much in order to develop a new instrument, as to see if SD is affecting the subject's responses. If it is not, then there is little to be concerned about; if so, though, there is little that can be done after the fact except to exercise caution in interpreting the results. Unfortunately, the correlations among the social desirability scales are low. Holden and Fekken (1989) found that the Jackson and Edwards scales correlated 0.71, but that the correlation between the Jackson and Crowne–Marlowe scales was only 0.27, and 0.26 between the Edwards and Crowne–Marlowe scales. They interpreted their factor analysis of these three scales to mean that the Jackson and Edwards scales measured 'a sense of own general capability', and the Crowne–Marlowe scale tapped 'interpersonal sensitivity'. Similar results were found by Paulhus (1983, 1984). He believes that his factor analysis of various scales indicates that the Edwards scale taps the more covert tendency of social desirability (what he calls 'self-deception'), while the Crowne–Marlowe scale comprises aspects of both self-deception and faking good (his term is 'impression management'). These findings would explain the relatively low correlation between the Crowne–Marlowe scale and the others.

This leaves the scale constructor in something of a quandary regarding which, if any, SD scale to use. Most people use the Crowne and Marlowe scale, probably more by habit and tradition than because of any superior psychometric qualities. Holden and Fekken's advice, which is reasonable in light of their results, is to use two indices: the Crowne–Marlowe scale and either the Jackson or the Edwards.

A second method to measure and reduce SD, used by McFarlane *et al.* (1981) in the development of their *Social Relations Scale*, is to administer the scale twice; once using the regular instructions to the subjects regarding its completion, and then asking them to fill it in as they would like things to be, or in the best of all possible worlds. This involved asking them first to list whom they talk to about issues that come up in their lives in various areas. A few weeks later (by which time they should have forgotten their original responses), they were asked to complete it 'according to what you consider to be good or ideal circumstances'. If the scores on any item did not change from the first to the second administration, it was assumed that its original answer was dictated more by SD than by the true state of affairs (or was at the 'ceiling' and could not detect any improvement). In either case, the item failed to satisfy at least one desired psychometric property, and was eliminated.

The term 'faking good' is most often applied to an intentional and deliberate approach by the person in responding to personality inventories. An analogous bias in responding to items on questionnaires is called 'prestige bias' (Oppenheim 1966). To judge from responses on questionnaires, nobody watches game shows or soap operas on TV, despite their obvious popularity; everyone watches only educational and cultural programmes. Their only breaks from these activities are to attend concerts, visit museums, and brush their teeth four or five times each day. (One can only wonder why the concert halls are empty and dentists' waiting rooms are full.)

Whyte (1956, p. 197), only half in jest, gave some advice to business people who had to take personality tests in order for them to advance up the company ladder. He wrote that, in order to select the best reply to a question, the person should repeat to himself:

- I loved my father and my mother, but my father a little bit more.
- I like things pretty well the way they are.
- I never much worry about anything.
- I don't care for books or music much.
- I love my wife and children.
- I don't let them get in the way of company work.

Since faking good and the prestige bias are more volitional than social desirability, they are easier to modify through instructions and careful wording of the items. The success of these tactics, though, is still open to question.

Deviation and faking bad

The opposite of socially desirable responding and faking good are *deviation* and *faking bad*. These latter two phenomena have been less studied than their positive counterparts, and no scales to assess them are in wide use. Deviation is a concept introduced by Berg (1967) to explain (actually, simply to name) the tendency to respond to test items with deviant responses. As is the case for faking good, faking bad occurs primarily within the context of personality assessment, although this may happen any time a person feels he or she may avoid an unpleasant situation (such as the military draft) by looking bad.

Both SD (or perhaps faking good) and deviance (or faking bad) occur together in an interesting phenomenon called the 'hello–goodbye' effect. Before an intervention, a person may present himself in as bad a light as possible, thereby hoping to qualify for the program, and impressing the staff with the seriousness of his problems. At termination, he may want to 'please' the staff with his improvement, and so may minimize any problems. The result is to make it appear that there has been improvement when none has occurred, or to magnify any effects which did occur. This effect was originally described in psychother-apy research, but it may arise whenever a subject is assessed on two occasions, with some intervention between the administrations of the scale.

Three techniques have been proposed to minimize the effects of these differ-ent biases. One method is to try to disguise the intent of the test, so the subject does not know what is actually being looked for. Rotter's scale to measure locus of control (Rotter 1966), for example, is called the *Personal Reaction Inventory*, a vague title which conveys little about the purpose of the instrument. (But then again, neither does 'locus of control'.)

However, this deception is of little use if the content of the items themselves reveals the objective of the scale. Thus, the second method consists of using 'subtle' items, ones where the respondent is unaware of the specific trait or behaviour being tapped. The item may still have face validity, since the respon-dent could feel that the question is fair and relevant; however, its actual rel-evance may be to some trait other than that assumed by the answerer (Holden and Jackson 1979). For example, the item, 'I would enjoy racing motorcycles' may appear to measure preferences for spending one's leisure time, while in fact it may be on an index of risk-taking. The difficulty with this technique, though, is that the psychometric properties of subtle items are usually poorer than those of obvious ones, and often do not measure the traits for which they were originally intended (Burkhart *et al.* 1976; Jackson 1971).

The third method of minimizing social desirability bias, especially regarding illegal, immoral, or embarrassing behaviours, is called the *random response tech-nique* (Warner 1965). In the most widely used of many variants of the technique, the respondent is handed a card containing two items; one neutral and one sensi-tive. For example, the questions can be:

A. I own a VCR.

B. I have used street drugs within the past six months.

The respondent is also given a device which randomly selects an A or a B. This can be as simple as a coin, or a spinner mounted on a card divided into two zones, each labelled with one of the letters. He or she is told to flip the coin (or spin the arrow), and truthfully answer whichever item is indicated; the inter-viewer is not to know *which* question has been selected, only the response.

In practice, only a portion of the respondents are given these items; the remaining subjects are asked the neutral question directly in order to determine the prevalence of 'True' responses to it in the sample. When two or more such items are used, half of the group will be given the random response technique on half of the questions, and asked about the neutral stems for the remaining items; while this would be reversed for the second half of the sample. An alternative is to use a neutral item where the true prevalence is well known, such as the pro-portion of families owning two cars or with three children. Of course, the scale developer must be quite sure that the sample is representative of the population on which the prevalence figures were derived.

With this information, the proportion of people answering 'true' to the sensitive item (p_s) can be estimated using the equation

$$p_s = [p_t - (1 - P)\, p_d]/P$$

where p_t is the proportion of people who answered 'true', p_d is the proportion saying 'true' to the neutral item on direct questioning, and P is the probability of selecting the sensitive item.

The variance of p_s is

$$Var\,(p_s) = \frac{p_t\,(1 - p_t)}{nP^2}$$

and the estimated standard error is the square root of this.

The probability of selecting the sensitive item (P) is 50 per cent using a coin toss, but can be modified with other techniques. For example, the two zones on the spinner can be divided so that A covers only 30 per cent and B 70 per cent. Another modification uses two colours of balls drawn from an urn; here, the proportion of each colour (representing each stem) can be set at other than 50 per cent. The closer P is to 1.0, the smaller the sample size needed to get an accurate estimate of p_s, but the technique begins to resemble direct questioning, and anonymity becomes jeopardized.

One difficulty with this form of the technique is the necessity to think of neutral questions and estimate their prevalence. An alternative approach, proposed by Greenberg *et al.* (1969), is to divide the spinner into three zones, or use three colours of balls. The subject is required to (1) answer the sensitive question truthfully if the spinner lands in zone A (or colour A is chosen); (2) say 'yes' if the spinner points to zone B; or (3) say 'no' if it ends up in zone C. The estimates of p_s and its variance are the same as in the previous case. Although this variant eliminates one problem, it leads to another; some people told to answer 'yes' actually respond 'no' in order to avoid appearing to have engaged in an illegal or embarrassing act.

Another difficulty with the original Warner technique and its variants is that they are limited to asking questions with only dichotomous answers; 'yes – no' or 'true – false'. Greenberg *et al.* (1971) modified this so that both the sensitive and the neutral questions ask for numerical answers, such as:

A. How many times during the past year have you slept with someone who isn't your spouse?
B. How many children do you have?

In this case, the estimated mean of the sensitive item (μ_s) is:

$$\mu_s = \frac{(1 - P_1)\, \bar{z}_1 - (1 - P_2)\, \bar{z}_2}{P_1 - P_2}$$

with variance

$$Var\,(\mu_s) = \frac{(1 - P_2)^2 \left(\dfrac{s_1^2}{n_1}\right) + (1 - P_1)^2 \left(\dfrac{s_2^2}{n_2}\right)}{(P_1 - P_2)^2}$$

where $\bar{z}_1$ is the mean for sample 1, n_1 is its sample size, s_1^2 the variance of $\bar{z}_1$ for sample 1, and P_1 the probability of having chosen question A. The terms with the subscript '2' are for a second sample, which is needed to determine the mean value of question B. Other variations on this theme are discussed by Scheers (1992).

The advantage of the random response technique is that it gives a more accurate estimate of the true prevalence of these sensitive behaviours than does direct questioning. For example, nine times as many women reported having had an abortion when asked with the random response method as compared with traditional questioning (Shimizu and Bonham 1978). However, there are some penalties associated with this procedure. First, it is most easily done in face-to-face interviews, although it is possible over the telephone. Second, since it is not known which subjects responded to each stem, the answers cannot be linked to other information from the questionnaire. Third, the calculated prevalence depends upon three estimates: the proportion of subjects responding to the sensitive item; the proportion answering 'true'; and the proportion of people who respond 'true' to the neutral stem. Since each of these is measured with error, a much larger sample size is required to get stable estimates.

Yea-saying or acquiescence

Yea-saying, also called *acquiescence bias*, is the tendency to give positive responses, such as 'true', 'like', 'often', or 'yes', to a question (Couch and Keniston 1960). At its most extreme, the person responds in this way irrespective of the content of the item, so that even mutually contradictory statements are endorsed. Thus, the person may respond 'true' to two items like 'I always take my medication on time,' and 'I often forget to take my pills.' At the opposite end of the spectrum are the 'nay-sayers.' It is believed that this tendency is more or less normally distributed, so that relatively few people are at the extremes, but that many people exhibit this trait to lesser degrees.

The amount that has been written about yea– and nay-saying can literally fill volumes. Despite this, there is still considerable controversy whether or not it actually exists. Rorer (1965), for example, acknowledges that some people are more prone to answer 'true' than 'false', but maintains that this tendency exists only on tests which tap a person's knowledge (what he calls 'examinations'), and when the person is ignorant of the correct answer. Insofar as personality tests are concerned, though, he states that his review of the extensive literature failed to show a content-free tendency to agree or disagree with any statement. Just as vehemently, Jackson (1967) and Messick (1967) argue that acquiescence (and its opposite) have been amply demonstrated, and pose real threats to test construction. The safest path to take is to assume that it exists, and try to minimize it.

No specific scales have been developed to measure yea-saying or nay-saying. Rather, some people (see for example Phillips and Clancy 1970) simply count the number of items on a scale answered positively or negatively by each subject. The usual way to correct for this potential bias is to have an equal number of items keyed in the positive and negative directions. A scale for compliance with medication, then, would be randomly divided so that 'true' on half of the items would reflect compliance, as would 'false' on the remaining ones. As mentioned in Chapter 5, however, the items should be balanced with respect to how they are *keyed*, but negatively *worded* items should be avoided.

End-aversion, positive skew, and halo

In addition to the distortions already mentioned, scales which are scored on a continuum, such as visual analogue and Likert scales, are prone to other types of biases. These include end-aversion bias, positive skew, and the halo effect.

End-aversion bias

End-aversion bias, which is also called the *central tendency bias*, refers to the reluctance of some people to use the extreme categories of a scale. It is based in part on people's difficulty in making absolute judgements, since situations without mitigating or extenuating circumstances rarely occur. The problem is similar to the one some people have in responding to 'true—false' items; they often want to say, 'It all depends,' or 'Most of the time, but not always.' The effect of this bias is to reduce the range of possible responses. Thus, if the extremes of a five-point Likert scale are labelled 'always' and 'never,' an end-aversion bias would render this a three-point scale, with the resulting loss of sensitivity and reliability.

There are two ways of dealing with the end-aversion bias. The first is to avoid absolute statements at the end-points; using 'almost never' and 'almost always' instead of 'never' and 'always.' The problem with this approach is that data may be thrown away; some people may *want* to respond with absolutes, but not allowing them to dilutes their answers with less extreme ones. The advantage is a greater probability that all categories will be used.

The second, and opposite, tack is to include 'throw away' categories at the ends. If the aim is to have a seven-point scale, then nine alternatives are provided, with the understanding that the extreme boxes at the ends will rarely be checked, but are there primarily to serve as anchors. This more or less ensures that all seven categories of interest will be used, but may lead to the problem of devising more adjectives if each box is labelled.

Positive skew

It often happens, though, that the responses are not evenly distributed over the range of alternatives, but show a positive *skew* toward the favourable end. This situation is most acute when a rating scale is used to evaluate students or staff.

For example, Linn (1979) found that the mean score on a five-point scale was 4.11 rather than 3.00, and the scores ranged between 3.30 and 4.56—the lower half of the scale was never used. Similarly, Cowles and Kubany (1959) asked raters to determine if a student was in the lower one-fifth, top one-fifth, or middle three-fifths of the class. Despite these explicit instructions, 31 per cent were assigned to the top fifth and only 5 per cent to the bottom one-fifth.

This may reflect the feeling that since these students survived the hurdles of admission into university and then into professional school, the 'average' student is really quite exceptional. It is then difficult to shift sets, so that 'average' is relative to the other people in the normative group, rather than the general population.

The effect of skew is to produce a *ceiling effect*; since most of the marks are clustered in only a few boxes at one extreme, the scores are very near the top of the scale. This means that it is almost impossible to detect any improvement, or to distinguish among various grades of excellence.

A few methods have been proposed to counteract this bias, all based on the fact that 'average' need not be in the middle. Since no amount of instruction or training appears to be able to shake an evaluator's belief that the average person under his or her supervision is far above average, the aim of a scale is then to differentiate among degrees of excellence. Using a traditional Likert scale, like:

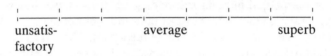

will result in most of the scores bunching in the three right-most boxes (or two, if an end-aversion is also present). However, we can shift the centre to look like this:

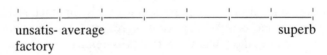

This gives the evaluator five boxes above average, rather than just three.

Another strategy is to capitalize on the fact that the truly superb students or employees need little feedback, except to continue doing what they have been all along, while the unsatisfactory ones are readily apparent to all evaluators even without scales. Rather, we should use the scale to differentiate among the majority of people who fall between these extremes. In this situation, the middle is expanded, at the expense of the ends:

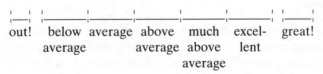

Note that this version clearly distinguishes the extremes, and offsets 'average'; many other variations on this theme are possible, reflecting the needs and philosophies of the program.

Halo

Halo is a phenomenon first recognized 80 years ago (Wells 1907), whereby judgements made on individual aspects of a person's performance are influenced by the rater's overall impression of the person. Thorndike (1920), who named this effect, gave what is still the best description of it: 'The judge seems intent on reporting his final opinion of the strength, weakness, merit, or demerit of the personality as a whole, rather than on giving as discriminating a rating as possible for each separate characteristic' (p. 447). For example, if a resident is well regarded by a staff physician, then the resident will be evaluated highly in all areas. Conversely, a resident who is felt to be weak in clinical skills, for example, can do no right, and will receive low scores in all categories. To some degree, this reflects reality; people who are good at one thing tend to do well in related areas. Also, many of the individual categories are dependent upon similar traits or behaviours: the ability to establish rapport with patients likely is dependent on the same skills that are involved in working with nurses and other staff. Cooper (1981) refers to this real correlation among categories as 'true halo'.

However, the ubiquity of this phenomenon and the very high intercorrelations among many different categories indicate that more is going on: what Cooper calls 'illusory halo', and what we commonly refer to when we speak of the 'halo effect'. There have been many theories proposed to explain illusory halo, but many simply boil down to the fact that raters are unable to evaluate people along more than a few dimensions. Very often, one global, summary rating scale about the person conveys as much information as do the individual scales about each aspect of the person's performance.

Many of the techniques proposed to minimize illusory halo involve factors other than the scale itself, such as the training of raters, basing the evaluations on larger samples of behaviour, and using more than one evaluator (e.g. Cooper 1981). The major aspect of scale design which may reduce this effect is the use of behaviourally-anchored ratings (BARs); instead of simply stating 'below average', for example, concrete examples are used, either as part of the descriptors themselves, or on a separate instruction page (e.g. Streiner 1985). This gives the raters concrete meaning for each level on the scale, reducing the subjective element and increasing agreement among raters.

Framing

Another bias, which particularly affects econometric scaling methods, is called *framing* (Kahneman and Tversky 1984). The name refers to the fact that the person's choice between two alternative states depends on how these states are framed. For example, consider the situation where an outbreak of influenza is expected to kill 600 people in the country. The subject must choose between two programs:

Program A: 200 people will be saved.
Program B: There is a one-third probability that 600 people will be saved, and two-thirds that nobody will be saved.

Nearly 75 per cent of subjects prefer Program A—assurance that 200 people will be saved—rather than the situation which offers the possibility that everyone could be saved, but at the risk of saving no one. Now consider presenting the same situation, but offering two different programs:

Program C: 400 people will die.
Program D: There is a one-third probability that nobody will die, and two-thirds that 600 will die.

Programs A and C are actually the same, as are B and D; all that differs is how the situations are presented (or 'framed'). In A, the number of survivors is explicitly stated, and the number who die (400) is implicit; this is reversed in C, where the number who die is given, but not the number who live. From a purely arithmetic point of view, the proportion of people opting for C, then, should be similar to those who choose A. In fact, over 75 per cent select program D rather than C, the exact reverse of the first situation.

Kahneman and Tversky explain these seemingly contradictory results by postulating that people are 'risk averse' when gain is involved and 'risk takers' in loss situations. That is, when offered the possibility of a gain (saving lives, winning a bet, and so on), people tend to take the safer route of being sure they gain something rather than the riskier alternative of perhaps getting much more, but possibly losing everything. In loss situations, though, such as choosing between Programs C and D, people will gamble on minimizing their losses (although there is the risk that they can lose everything), rather than taking the certain situation that they will lose something.

The problem that this poses for the designer of questionnaires is that the manner in which a question is posed can affect the results that are obtained. For example, if the researchers were interested in physicians' attitudes toward a new operation or drug, they may get very different answers if they said that the incidence of morbidity was 0.1 per cent, as opposed to saying that there was a 99.9 per cent chance that nothing untoward would occur.

In conclusion, the safest strategy for the test developer is to assume that all of these biases are operative, and take the necessary steps to minimize them whenever possible.

References

Anastasi, A. (1982). *Psychological testing* (5th edn). Macmillan, New York.
Berg, I. A. (1967). The deviation hypothesis: A broad statement of its assumptions and

postulates. In *Response set in personality assessment* (ed. I. A. Berg) pp. 146–90. Aldine, Chicago.

Burkhart, B. R., Christian, W. L., and Gynther, M. D. (1976). Item subtlety and faking on the MMPI: A paradoxical relationship. *Journal of Personality Assessment*, **42**, 76–80.

Cooper, W. H. (1981). Ubiquitous halo. *Psychological Bulletin*, **90**, 218–44.

Couch, A. and Keniston, K. (1960). Yeasayers and naysayers: Agreeing response set as a personality variable. *Journal of Abnormal and Social Psychology*, **60**, 151–74.

Cowles, J. T. and Kubany, A. J. (1959). Improving the measurement of clinical performance in medical students. *Journal of Clinical Psychology*, **15**, 139–42.

Crowne, D. P. and Marlowe, D. (1960). A new scale of social desirability independent of psychopathology. *Journal of Consulting Psychology*, **24**, 349–54.

Edwards, A. L. (1957). *The social desirability variable in personality assessments and research*. Dryden, New York.

Greenberg, B. C., Abul-Ela, A., Simmons, W., and Horvitz, D. (1969). The unrelated question randomized response model: Theoretical framework. *Journal of the American Statistical Association*, **64**, 520–39.

Greenberg, B. C., Kuebler, R. R., Abernathy, J. R., and Horvitz, D. G. (1971). Application of the randomized response technique in obtaining quantitative data. *Journal of the American Statistical Association*, **66**, 243–50.

Holden, R. R. and Fekken, G. C. (1989). Three common social desirability scales: Friends, acquaintances, or strangers? *Journal of Research in Personality*, **23**, 180–91.

Holden, R. R. and Jackson, D. N. (1979). Item subtlety and face validity in personality assessment. *Journal of Consulting and Clinical Psychology*, **47**, 459–68.

Jackson, D. N. (1967). Acquiescence response styles: Problems of identification and control. In *Response set in personality assessment* (ed. I. A. Berg) pp. 71–114. Aldine, Chicago.

Jackson, D. N. (1970). A sequential system for personality scale development. In *Current topics in clinical and community psychology* (ed. C. D. Spielberger), Vol. 2 pp. 61–96. Academic Press, New York.

Jackson, D. N. (1971). The dynamics of structured personality tests: 1971. *Psychological Review*, **78**, 229–48.

Jackson, D. N. (1984). *Personality Research Form manual*. Research Psychologists Press, Port Huron, MI.

Kahneman, D. and Tversky, A. (1984). Choices, values, and frames. *American Psychologist*, **39**, 341–50.

Krosnick, J. A. (1991). Response strategies for coping with the cognitive demands of attitude measures in surveys. *Applied Cognitive Psychology*, **5**, 213–36.

Linn, L. (1979). Interns' attitudes and values as antecedents of clinical performance. *Journal of Medical Education*, **54**, 238–40.

McFarlane, A. H., Neale, K. A., Norman, G. R., Roy, R. G., and Streiner, D. L. (1981). Methodological issues in developing a scale to measure social support. *Schizophrenia Bulletin*, **7**, 90–100.

Messick, S. J. (1967). The psychology of acquiescence: An interpretation of the research evidence. In *Response set in personality assessment* (ed. I. A. Berg) pp. 115–45. Aldine, Chicago.

Oppenheim, A. N. (1966). *Questionnaire design and attitude measurement*. Heinemann, London.

Paulhus, D. L. (1983). Sphere-specific measures of perceived control. *Journal of Personality and Social Psychology*, **44**, 1253–65.

Paulhus, D. L. (1984). Two-component models of socially desirable responding. *Journal of Personality and Social Psychology*, **46**, 598–609.

Phillips, D. L. and Clancy, K. J. (1970). Response biases in field studies of mental illness. *American Sociological Review*, **35**, 503–15.

Rorer, L. G. (1965). The great response-style myth. *Psychological Bulletin*, **63**, 129–56.

Rotter, J. (1966). Generalized expectancies for internal versus external control of reinforcement. *Psychological Monographs: General and Applied*, **80** (1, Whole No. 609).

Scheers, N. J. (1992). A review of randomized response techniques. *Measurement and Evaluation in Counseling and Development*, **25**, 27–41.

Shimizu, I. M. and Bonham, G. S. (1978). Randomized response technique in a national survey. *Journal of the American Statistical Association*, **73**, 35–9.

Simon, H. A. (1957). *Models of man*. Wiley, New York.

Streiner, D. L. (1985). Global rating scales. In *Assessing clinical competence* (eds. V. R. Neufeld and G. R. Norman), pp. 119–41. Springer, New York.

Sudman, S. and Bradburn, N. M. (1982). *Asking questions: A practical guide to questionnaire design*. Jossey-Bass, San Francisco.

Thorndike, E. L. (1920). A constant error in psychological ratings. *Journal of Applied Psychology*, **4**, 25–9.

Tourangeau, R. (1984). Cognitive sciences and survey methods. In *Cognitive aspects of survey methodology: Building a bridge between disciplines* (eds. T. Jabine, M. Straf, J. Tanur, and R. Tourangeau) pp. 73–100. National Academy Press, Washington DC.

Warner, S. L. (1965). Randomized response: A survey technique for eliminating evasive answer bias. *Journal of the American Statistical Association*, **60**, 63–9.

Wells, F. L. (1907). A statistical study of literary merit. *Archives of Psychology*, **1**(7).

Whyte, W. H., Jr. (1956). *The organization man*. Simon and Schuster, New York.

7

From items to scales

Some scales consist of just one item, such as a visual analogue scale, on which a person may rate his or her pain on a continuum from 'no pain at all' to 'the worst imaginable pain'. However, the more usual and desirable approach is to have a number of items to assess a single underlying characteristic. This then raises the issue of how we combine the individual items into a scale, and then express the final score in the most meaningful way.

By far the easiest solution is to simply add the scores on the individual items and leave it at that. In fact, this is the approach used by many scales. The *Beck Depression Inventory* (BDI; Beck *et al.* 1961), for instance, consists of 21 items, each scored on a 0–3 scale, so the final score can range between 0 and 63. This approach is conceptually and arithmetically simple, and makes few assumptions about the individual items; the only implicit assumption is that the items are equally important in contributing to the total score.

Since this approach is so simple, there must be something wrong with it. Actually, there are two potential problems. We say 'potential' because, as will be seen later, they may not be problems in certain situations. First, some items may be more important than others, and perhaps should make a larger contribution to the total score. Second, unlike the situation in measuring blood pressure, for example, where it is expected that each of the different methods should yield exactly the same answer, no one presumes that all scales tapping activities of daily living should give the same number at the end. Under these circumstances, it is difficult, if not impossible, to compare scores on different scales, since each uses a different metric. We shall examine both of these points in some more detail.

Weighting the items

Rather than simply adding up all of the items, a scale or index may be developed which 'weights' each item differently in its contribution to the total score. There are two general approaches to doing this, theoretical and empirical. In the former, a test constructor may feel that, based on his or her understanding of the field, there are some aspects of a trait that are crucial, and others which are still interesting, but perhaps less germane. It would make at least intuitive sense for the former to be weighted more heavily than the latter. For example, in assessing the recovery of a cardiac patient, his or her ability to return to work may be seen as more important than resumption of leisure-time activities. In this case, the scale developer may multiply, or weight, the score on items relating to the first set of activities by a factor which would reflect its greater importance. (Perhaps we should mention here that the term 'weight' is preferred by statisticians to the more commonly used 'weigh'.)

The empirical approach comes from the statistical theory of multiple regression. Very briefly, in multiple regression we try to predict a score (Y) from a number of independent items (Xs), and takes the form:

$$Y = \beta_0 + \beta_1 X_1 + \beta_2 X_2 + \ldots + \beta_k X_k$$

where β_0 is a constant, and $\beta_1 \ldots \beta_k$ are the 'beta weights' for the k items.

We choose the βs to maximize the predictive accuracy of the equation. There is one optimal set, and any other set of values will result in less accuracy. In the case of a scale, Y is the trait or behaviour we are trying to predict, and the Xs are the individual items. This would indicate that a weighting scheme for each item, empirically derived, would improve the accuracy of the total score (leaving aside for the moment the question of what we mean by 'accuracy').

One obvious penalty for this greater sophistication introduced by weighting is increased computation. Each item's score must be multiplied by a constant, and these then added together; a process which is more time-consuming and prone to error than treating all items equally (i.e. giving them all weights of 1).

The question then is whether the benefits outweigh the costs. The answer is that it all depends. Wainer's (1976) conclusion was that if we eliminate items with very small β weights (that is, those that contribute little to the overall accuracy anyway), then 'it don't make no nevermind' whether the other items are weighted or not.

This was demonstrated empirically by Lei and Skinner (1980), using the Holmes and Rahe (1967) *Social Readjustment Rating Scale* (SRRS). This checklist consists of events which may have occurred in the past six months, and weighted to reflect how much adjustment would be required to adapt to it. Lei and Skinner looked at four versions of the SRRS: using the original weights assigned by Holmes and Rahe; using simply a count of the number of items endorsed, which is the same as using weights of 1 for all items; using 'perturbed' weights, where they were randomly shuffled from one item to another; and randomly assigned weights, ranging between 1 and 100.

The life events scale would appear to be an ideal situation for using weights, since there is a 100-fold difference between the lowest and highest. On the surface, at least, this differential weighting makes sense, since it seems ridiculous to assign the same weight to the death of a spouse as to receiving a parking ticket. However, they found that the correlations among these four versions was 0.97. In other words, it did not matter whether original weights, random weights, or no weights were used; people who scored high on one variant scored high on all of the others, and similarly for people who scored at the low end. Similar results with the SRRS were found by Streiner *et al.* (1981).

Moreover, this finding is not peculiar to the SRRS; it has been demonstrated with a wide variety of personality and health status measures (e.g. Jenkinson 1991; Streiner *et al.* 1993). Indeed, Gulliksen (1950) derived an equation to predict how much (or rather, how little) item weighting will affect a scale's correlation with other measures, and hence its validity. The correlation (*R*) between the weighted and unweighted versions of a test is:

$$R = 1 - \left(\frac{1}{2\,K\bar{r}}\right)\left(\frac{s}{M}\right)^2$$

where *K* is the number of items in the scale,
    $\bar{r}$ is the average correlation among the *K* items,
    M is the average of the weights, and
    s is the standard deviation of the weights.

What this equation shows is that the correlation between the weighted and unweighted versions of the test is higher when (a) there are more items, (b) the average inter-item correlation is higher, and (c) the standard deviation of the weights is lower relative to their mean value. Empirical testing has shown that actual values are quite close to those predicted by the formula (Retzlaff *et al.* 1990; Streiner and Miller 1989).

To complicate matters, though, a very different conclusion was reached by Perloff and Persons (1988). They indicated that weighting can significantly increase the predictive ability of an index, and criticize Wainer's work because he limited his discussion to situations where the β weights were evenly distributed over the interval from 0.25 to 0.75, which they feel is an improbable situation.

So, what conclusion can we draw from this argument? The answer is far from clear. It would seem that when there are at least 40 items in a scale, differential weighting contributes relatively little, except added complexity for the scorer. With fewer than 40 items (20, according to Nunnally, 1970), weighting *may* have some effect. The other consideration is that if the scale is comprised of relatively homogeneous items, where the β weights will all be within a fairly narrow range, the effect of weighting may be minimal. However, if an index consists of unrelated items, as is sometimes the case with functional status measures, then it may be worthwhile to run a multiple regression analysis and determine empirically if this improves the predictive ability of the scale.

There are two forms of weighting that are more subtle than multiplying each item by a number, and are often unintended. The first is having a different number of items for various aspects of the trait being measured, and the second is including items which are highly correlated with one another. To illustrate the first point, assume we are devising a scale to assess childhood difficulties. In this instrument, we have one item tapping into problems associated with going to bed, and five items looking at disciplinary problems. This implicitly assigns more weight to the latter category, since its potential contribution to the total score can be five times as great as the first area. Even if the parents feel that putting the child to bed is more troublesome to them than the child's lack of discipline, the scale would be weighted in the opposite direction.

There are a few ways around this problem. First, the number of items tapping each component can be equal (which assumes that all aspects contribute equally), or proportional to the importance of that area. An item-by-item matrix can be used to verify this, as was discussed in Chapter 3. A second solution is to have sub-scales, each comprised of items in one area. The total for the sub-scale would be the number of items endorsed divided by the total number of items within the sub-scale (and perhaps multiplied by 10 or 100 to eliminate decimals). The scale total is then derived by adding up these transformed sub-scale scores. In this way, each sub-scale contributes equally to the total score, even though each sub-scale may consist of a different number of items.

The second form of implicit weighting is through correlated items. Using the same example of a scale for childhood problems, assume that the section on school-related difficulties includes the following items:

1. Is often late for school
2. Talks back to the teacher
3. Often gets into fights
4. Does not obey instructions
5. Ignores the teacher

If items 2, 4, and 5 are highly correlated, then getting a score on any one of them almost automatically leads to scores on the other two. Thus, these three items are likely measuring the same thing and, as such, constitute a sub-sub-scale, and lead to problems analogous to those found with the first form of subtle weighting. The same solutions can be used, as well as a third solution: eliminating two of the items. This problem is almost universal, since we expect items tapping the same trait to be correlated; just not *too* correlated.

Unlike explicit weighting, these two forms are often unintentional. If the effects are unwanted (as they often are), special care and pre-testing the instrument are necessary to ensure that they do not occur.

Multiplicative composite scores

The previous section focused on the situation in which each item was given the same weight, and the conclusion was that it is hardly ever worth the effort. In this section, we will discuss a seemingly similar case—where each item is given a different weight by different subjects—and come to a similar recommendation: don't do it unless it is unavoidable or you are prepared to pay the price in terms of increased sample size and complexity in analysing the results.

Multiplicative composite scores are those in which two values are multiplied together to yield one number. At first glance, this would seem to be a very useful manoeuvre with few drawbacks. Imagine, for example, that supervisors must rate interns on a form which lists a number of components, such as clinical skills, interpersonal skills, self-directed learning, and knowledge base. In any one rotation, the supervisor may have had ample opportunity to observe how the student performs in some of these areas, but may have had a more limited chance to see others. It would seem to make sense that we should ask the supervisor a second question for each component, 'How confident are you in this rating?'. Then, when the rating is multiplied by the confidence level, those areas in which the supervisor was more confident would make a greater contribution to the total score, and areas where the supervisor was not as confident would add less. Similarly, if you were devising a quality of life scale, it would seem sensible to multiply people's rating of how well or poorly they could perform some task by some other index which reflects the importance of that task for them. In that way, a person would not be penalized by being unable to do tasks which are done rarely or not at all (e.g. males are not too concerned about their inability to reach behind their back to do up their bra, nor females by the fact that they have difficulty shaving their faces each morning). Conversely, the total score on the scale would be greatly affected by the important tasks, thus making it easier to detect any changes in quality of life due to some intervention or over time.

The problem arises because multiplying two numbers together (i.e. creating a composite measure) affects the resulting total's correlation with another score. More importantly, even if the ratings are kept the same, but simply transformed from one weighting scheme to another (e.g. changed from a -3 to $+3$ system to a 1 to 7 point scheme), *the scale's correlation with another scale can alter dramatically*.

To illustrate this, imagine that we have an instrument with five items, where each item is scored along a 7-point Likert scale. These are then summed, to form a score (X) for each of five subjects. The items, and their sums, are shown in the second column of Table 7.1, the one labelled Item Score (X). If we correlate these five totals with some other measure, labelled Y in the Table, we find that the correlation is 0.927.

Next assume that each item is weighted for importance on a 7-point scale, with 1 indicating not at all important, and 7 extremely important (column 3 in Table 7.1). These scores are then multiplied by X, and the result, along with each subject's total, are shown in column 4. If we correlate these totals with the Ys, we find that the result is 0.681. Now comes the interesting part. Let us keep exactly the same weights for each person, but score them on a 7-point scale where not at all important is -3, and extremely important is $+3$; that is, we have done nothing more than subtract four points from each weight. The results of this are shown in the last two columns.

Has this changed anything? Amazingly, the results are drastically different. Instead of a correlation of $+0.681$, we now find that the correlation is -0.501. That is, by keeping the weights the same, and simply modifying the numbers assigned to each point on the scale, we have transformed a relatively high positive correlation into an almost equally high negative one. Other linear transfor-

Table 7.1   *The effects of changing weighting schemes*

Subject		Item Score (X)	Y	+1 to +7 Weighting		−3 to +3 Weighting	
				Weight	Total	Weight	Total
1		7		1	7	−3	−21
		5		2	10	−2	−10
		7		3	21	−1	−7
		6		4	24	0	0
		3		5	15	1	3
	Total	28	25		77		−35
2		1		6	6	2	2
		3		7	21	3	9
		1		1	1	−3	−3
		2		2	4	−2	−4
		4		3	12	−1	−4
	Total	11	13		44		0
3		3		4	12	0	0
		4		5	20	1	4
		5		6	30	2	10
		4		7	28	3	12
		3		1	3	−1	−3
	Total	19	18		93		23
4		5		2	10	−2	−10
		7		3	21	−1	−7
		6		4	24	0	0
		3		5	15	1	3
		2		6	12	2	4
	Total	23	26		82		−10
5		2		7	14	3	6
		3		1	3	−3	−9
		2		2	4	−2	−4
		4		3	12	−1	−4
		5		4	20	0	0
	Total	16	15		53		−11

mations of the weights can make the correlation almost any value in between (or even more extreme).

Why should this be? The mathematics of it are beyond the scope of this book (the interested reader should look at Evans (1991) for a complete explanation). A brief summary is that the correlation between X and Y, where X is a composite score, depends in part on the variance of the weight, the covariance between X and the weight, and the mean of the weight. Thus, a change which affects any of these factors, but especially the weight's mean, can drastically affect the magnitude and the sign of the correlation.

There is a way to overcome the problem, but it is a costly one in terms of sample size. The method is to use hierarchical regression; that is, where the predictor variables are put into the regression equation in stages, under the control of the investigator (see Norman and Streiner (1994) for a fuller explanation). In the first step, any covariates are forced into the model. In step two, the X variable and the weights are added as two additional variables. In the third step, the interaction (i.e. the multiplication) of X and the weight is forced in. Any significant increase in the multiple correlation from step 1 to step 2 would indicate that the variables add something to the prediction of Y. Then, the real test of the hypothesis is to see if the multiple correlation increases significantly between the second and third steps; if so, it would show that the interaction between X and the weight adds something over and above what the variables tell us separately. Of course, we can also break step 2 down, to see if the weights themselves increase the predictive power of the equation.

The cost is that, rather than having one predictor and one dependent variable (ignoring any covariates), we now have three predictors: X, the weighting factor, and the interaction between the two. If we want to maintain a ratio of at least 10 subjects for every predictor variable (Norman and Streiner 1994), this triples the required sample size. In the end, unless one's theory demands an interaction term, multiplicative composites should be avoided.

Transforming the final score

The second drawback with simply adding up the items to derive a total score is that each new scale is reported on a different metric, making comparisons among scales difficult. This may not pose a problem if you are working in a brand new area, and do not foresee comparing the results to any other test. However, few such areas exist, and in most cases it is desirable to see how a person did on two different instruments. For example, the *BDI*, as we have said, ranges between a minimum score of 0 and a maximum of 63; while a similar test, the *Self-Rating Depression Scale* (SRDS; Zung 1965), yields a total score between 25 and 100. How can we compare a score of 23 on the former with one of 68 on the latter? It is not easy when the scores are expressed as they are.

The problem is even more evident when a test is comprised of many subscales, each with a different number of items. Many personality tests, like the *16PF* (Cattell *et al.* 1970) or the *Personality Research Form* (Jackson 1984) are constructed in such a manner, as are intelligence tests like those developed by Wechsler (1981). The resulting 'profile' of scale scores, comparing their relative elevations, would be uninterpretable if each scale were measured on a different yardstick.

The solution to this problem involves *transforming* the raw score in some way in order to facilitate interpretation. In this section, we discuss three different methods: percentiles, standard and standardized scores, and normalized scores.

Percentiles

A *percentile* is the percentage of people who score below a certain value; the lowest score is at the 0th percentile, since nobody has a lower one, while the top score is at the 99th percentile. Nobody can be at the 100th percentile, since that implies that everyone, including that person, has a lower score, an obvious impossibility. In medicine, perhaps the most widely used example of scales expressed in percentiles are developmental height and weight charts. After a child has been measured, his height is plotted on a table for children the same age. If he is at the 50th percentile, that means that he is exactly average for his age; half of all children are taller and half are shorter.

To show how these are calculated, assume a new test has been given to a large, representative sample, which is called a 'normative' or 'reference' group. If the test is destined to be used commercially, 'large' often means 1000 or more carefully selected people; for more modest aims, 'large' can mean about 100 or so. The group should be chosen so that their scores span the range you would expect to find when you finally use the test. The next step is to put the scores in *rank order*, ranging from the highest to the lowest. For illustrative purposes, suppose the normative group consists of (a ridiculously small number) 20 people. The results would look something like Table 7.2.

Starting with the highest score, a 37 for Subject 5, 19 of the 20 scores are lower, so a raw score of 37 corresponds to the 95th percentile. Subject 3 has a raw score of 21; since 12 of the 20 scores are lower, he is at the 60th percentile (i.e. 12/20). A slight problem arises when there are ties, as with Subjects 17 and 8, or 19 and 14. If there are an odd number of ties, as exists for a score of 16, we take the middle person (Subject 20 in this case), and count the number of people below. Since there are six of them, a raw score of 16 is at the 30th percentile, and all three people then get this value. If there are an even number of ties, then you will be dealing with 'halves' of a person. Thus, 8.5 people have scores lower than 17, so it corresponds to the 42.5th percentile. We continue doing this for all scores, and then rewrite the table, putting in the percentiles corresponding to each score, as in Table 7.3.

The major advantage of percentiles is that most people, even those without any training in statistics or scale development, can readily understand them. How-

Table 7.2 *Raw scores for 20 subjects on a hypothetical test*

Subject	Score	Subject	Score
5	37	19	17
13	32	14	17
2	31	1	16
15	29	20	16
17	26	7	16
8	23	6	15
10	23	11	13
3	21	16	12
12	20	4	10
18	19	9	8

Table 7.3 *The raw scores converted to percentiles*

Subject	Score	Percentile	Subject	Score	Percentile
5	37	95	19	17	42.5
13	32	90	14	17	42.5
2	31	85	1	16	35
15	29	80	20	16	35
17	26	75	7	16	35
8	23	67.5	6	15	25
10	23	67.5	11	13	20
3	21	60	16	12	10
12	20	55	4	10	5
18	18	50	9	8	0

ever, there are a number of difficulties with this approach. One problem is readily apparent in Table 7.3; unless you have many scores, there can be fairly large jumps between the percentile values of adjacent scores. Also, it is possible that in a new sample, some people may have scores higher or lower than those in the normative group, especially if it was small and not carefully chosen. This makes interpretation of these more extreme scores problematic at best. Third, since percentiles are ordinal data, they should not be analysed using parametric statistics; means and standard deviations derived from percentiles are not legitimate.

A fourth difficulty with percentiles is a bit more subtle, but just as insidious. The distribution of percentile scores is rectangular. However, the distribution of raw test scores usually resembles a normal, or bell-shaped, curve, with most of the values clustered around the mean, and progressively fewer ones as we move out to the extremes. As a result, small differences in the middle range become exaggerated, and large differences in the tails are truncated. For example, a score of 16 corresponds to the 35th percentile, while a score just two points higher is at the 50th percentile. By contrast, a five-point difference, from 32 to 37, results in just a five-point spread in the percentiles.

Standard and standardized scores

To get around these problems with percentiles, a more common approach is to use *standard scores*. The formula to transform raw scores to standard scores is

$$z = \frac{X - \bar{X}}{SD}$$

where X is the total score for an individual, $\bar{X}$ is the mean score of the sample, and SD is the sample's standard deviation.

This 'transforms' the scale to have a mean of 0 and a standard deviation of 1, so the individual scores are expressed in standard deviation units. Moreover, since the transformation is linear, the distribution of the raw scores (ideally normal) is preserved. For example, the mean of the 20 scores in the table is 20.0, and the standard deviation is 7.75. We can convert Subject 5's score of 37 into a z-score by putting these numbers into the formula. When we do this, we find

$$z = \frac{37 - 20}{7.75} = 2.19.$$

That is, his score of 37 is slightly more than two standard deviations above the mean on this scale. Similarly, a raw score of 12 yields a z-score of -1.55, showing that this person's score is about one and a half standard deviations below the group mean.

If all test scores were expressed in this way, then we could compare results across them quite easily. Indeed, we can use this technique on raw scores from different tests, as long as we have the means and standard deviations of the tests. Then, if we received scores on two tests given to a patient at two different times, and purportedly measuring the same thing, we can see if there has been any change by transforming both of them to z-scores. As an example, we can now answer the question, how does a score of 23 on the *BDI* compare with 68 on the *SRDS*? The mean and SD of the Beck are 11.3 and 7.7, and they are 52.1 and 10.5 for the Zung. Putting the raw scores into the equation with their respective means and SDs, we find that 23 on the Beck corresponds to a z-score of 1.52, and 65 on the Zung yields a z-score of 1.51. So, although the raw scores are very different, they probably reflect similar degrees of depression.

In real life, though, we are not used to seeing scores ranging from about -3.0 to $+3.0$; we are more accustomed to positive numbers only, and whole ones at

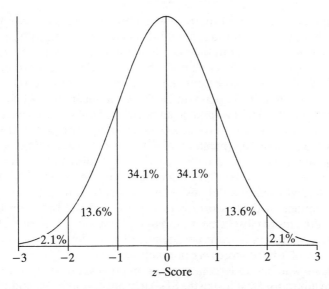

Fig. 7.1. The normal curve.

that. Very often, then, we take a second step and transform the z-score into what is called a *standardized* or *T-score*, by using the formula:

$$T = \bar{X}' + z(\mathrm{SD}')$$

where $\bar{X}'$ is the new mean that we want the test to have, SD$'$ is the desired standard deviation, and z is the original z-score.

We can also go directly from the raw scores to the T-scores by combining this equation with that for the z-score transformation, in which case we get

$$T = \bar{X}' + \frac{(\mathrm{SD}')\,(X - \bar{X})}{\mathrm{SD}}$$

A standardized or T-score is simply a z-score with a new mean and standard deviation, chosen relatively arbitrarily, and depending on custom, tradition, or just whim. For example, many personality tests use a mean of 50 and a standard deviation of 10 by convention; while the national tests for admission to university, graduate school, or professional programs use a mean of 500 and an SD of 100. Intelligence tests, for the most part, have a mean of 100 and an SD of 15. If we were developing a new IQ test, we would give it to a large normative sample and then transform each possible total raw score into a z-score. Then, setting $\bar{X}'$ to be 100 and SD$'$ to be 15, we would translate each z-score into its equivalent T-score. The result would be a new test, whose scores are directly comparable to those from older IQ tests.

The z- and T-scores do more than simply compare the results on two different tests. Like percentiles, they allow us to see where a person stands in relation to everybody else. If we assume that the scores on the test are fairly normally distributed, then we use the normal curve to determine what proportion of people score higher and lower. As a brief review, a normal curve looks like Figure 7.1. Most of the scores are clustered around the mean of the test, with progressively fewer scores as we move out to the tails. By definition, 50 per cent of the scores fall below the mean, and 50 per cent above; while 68 per cent are between -1 and $+1$ SD. That means that 84 per cent of scores fall below 1 SD—the 50 per cent below the mean plus 34 per cent between the mean and $+1$ SD. To use a concrete example, the *MCAT* has a mean of 500 and a standard deviation of 100. So, 68 per cent of the people have scores between 400 and 600, and 84 per cent have scores lower than 600 (meaning that 16 per cent have higher scores). We can look up other values in a table of the normal distribution, which can be found in most statistics books. This is an extremely useful property of z- and T-scores, which is why many widely-used tests report their final scores in this way. Another advantage of these scores is that, since they are based on the normal curve, they often more closely meet the assumptions of parametric statistics than do either raw scores or percentiles, although it is not safe to automatically assume that standardized scores *are* normally distributed.

Any clinician who has undergone the painful process of having to re-learn normal values of laboratory tests using the SI system must wonder why standard scores are not used in the laboratory. Indeed, the problem is twofold: switching from one measurement system to another; and different values of 'normal' within each system. For example, the normal range for fasting plasma glucose used to be between 70 and 110 mg per cent, and was 1.1–4.1 ng ml^{-1} h^{-1} for plasma renin. In SI units, these same values are 3.9–6.1 mmol l^{-1} for glucose, and 0.30–1.14 ng l^{-1} s^{-1} for renin. Think how much easier life would be if the results of all these diverse tests could be expressed in a common way, such as standard or standardized scores.

Normalized scores

In order to ensure that standard and standardized scores are normally distributed, we can use other transformations which normalize the raw scores. One of the most widely used ones is the *normalized standard score*. Returning to Table 7.3, we take one further step, transforming the percentiles into standard scores from a table of the normal curve. For example, the 95th percentile corresponds to a normalized standard score of 1.65; the 90th percentile to a score of 1.29, and so on. As with non-normalized standard scores, we can, if we wish, convert these to *standardized*, normalized scores, with any desired mean and standard deviation. In Table 7.4, we have added two more columns; the first showing the transformation from percentiles to normalized standard (z) scores, and then to normalized standardized (T) scores, using a mean of 100 and a standard deviation of 10.

Establishing cut points

Receiver Operating Characteristic curves

Although we have argued throughout this book that continuous measures are preferable to categorical ones, there are times when it is necessary to use a continuous

Table 7.4 *Percentiles transformed into normalized standard standardized scores*

Subject	Score	Percentile	Normalized standard score (z)	Normalized standardized score (T)
5	37	95	1.65	116.5
13	32	90	1.29	112.9
2	31	85	1.04	110.4
15	29	80	0.84	108.4
17	26	75	0.67	106.7
8	23	67.5	0.45	104.5
10	23	67.5	0.45	104.5
3	21	60	0.25	102.5
12	20	55	0.13	101.3
18	18	50	0.00	100.0
19	17	42.5	−0.19	98.1
14	17	42.5	−0.19	98.1
1	16	35	−0.39	96.1
20	16	35	−0.39	96.1
7	16	35	−0.39	96.1
6	15	25	−0.67	93.3
11	13	20	−0.84	91.6
16	12	10	−1.29	87.1
4	10	5	−1.65	83.5
9	8	0	−3.00	70.0

scale in order to predict a dichotomous outcome. For example, blood pressure (which is continuous) is taken to determine whether or not a person should be placed on some regimen (dichotomous), or a score on the *Beck Depression Inventory* is used to indicate the presence or absence of clinical depression. The problem then becomes determining the best cut-off score to use on the scale in order to make this discrimination.

The technique for establishing the optimal cut point is derived from the early days of radar and sonar detection in the Second World War (Peterson *et al.* 1954), and the name still reflects that—Receiver Operating Characteristic (ROC) curve. As we increase the sensitivity of the radio, we pick up both the sound we want to hear as well as background static. Initially, the signal increases faster than the noise. After some point, though, a cross-over is reached, where the noise grows faster than the signal. The optimal setting is where we detect the largest ratio of signal to noise. This technique was later applied to the psychological area of the ability of humans to detect the presence or absence of signals (Tanner and Swets 1954), and then to the ability of tests to detect the presence or absence of a state or disease.

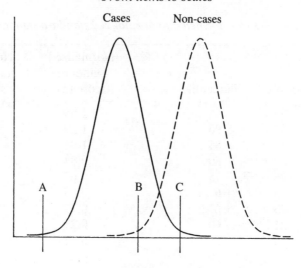

Fig. 7.2. Effects of different cut points.

Table 7.5 A 2×2 table for calculating sensitivity and specificity

		Gold Standard	
		Case	Non-case
New test	Case	A	B
	Non-case	C	D

In the assessment arena, the 'signal' is the number of actual cases of hypertension or depression detected by our scale; the 'noise' is the number of non-cases erroneously labelled as cases; and the analogue of amplification is the cut point of our new scale. If we use something like a quality of life scale, where lower scores indicate more problems, a very low cut-off score (Line A in Figure 7.2) will pick up few true cases, and also make few false positive errors. As we increase the cutting score (Line B), we hope we will pick up true cases faster than false ones. Above some optimal value, though, we will continue to detect more true cases, but at the cost of mislabelling many non-cases as cases (Line C). The task is to find this optimal value on our scale.

We begin by constructing a 2 × 2 table, as in Table 7.5. Cell A contains the number of actual cases (as determined by the dichotomous gold standard) who are labelled as cases by our new scale (the 'true positives'), while in Cell B are the non-cases erroneously labelled as cases by the test ('false positives'). Similarly, Cell C has the false negatives, and Cell D the true negatives. From this table, we can derive two necessary statistics: the *sensitivity* and the *specificity* of the test. Sensitivity (which is also called the *true positive rate*) is defined as A/(A + C); that is, is the test 'sensitive' in detecting a disorder when it is actually present? Specificity (or the *true negative rate*) is D/(B + D); is the test specific to this disorder, or is it elevated by other ones too?

To construct an ROC curve, we determine these two values for each possible cut point. Let us assume that we test 500 cases and 500 controls (non-cases) with our new test, which has a total score which could range from 10 to 20. The first row of our first table would contain all the people who had scores of 10, and the second row scores of 11 through 20; the first row of the second table would have scores of 10 and 11, and the second row 12 and higher; and so on, until the last table, where the top row would have all people with scores up to 19, and the bottom row those with a score of 20. (In order to make the graph start and end at one of the axes, we usually add two other tables; one in which everyone has a score above the cut point, and one where they all have scores below it.) The first few tables are shown in the top part of Table 7.6, and a summary of all 12 tables in the lower half. We then make a graph where the *X*–axis is 1 *minus* the specificity (i.e. the false positive rate), and the *Y*–axis is the sensitivity (also called the true positive rate), as in Figure 7.3.

The diagonal line which runs from point (0,0) in the lower left hand corner to (1,1) in the upper right reflects the characteristics of a test with no discriminating ability. The better a test is in dividing cases from non-cases, the closer it will approach the upper left hand corner. So, Test A in Figure 7.3 (which is based on the data in Table 7.6) is a better discriminator than Test B. The cut point which minimizes the overall number of errors (false positive and false negative) is the score which is closest to that corner. An index of the 'goodness' of the test is the area under the curve, which is usually abbreviated as D'. A non-discriminating test (one which falls on the diagonal) has an area of 0.5, and a perfect test has an area of 1.0. (If a test falls below the line, and has an area less than 0.5, then it is performing worse than chance; you would do better to simply go with the prevalence of the disorder in labelling people, rather than using the test results.) It is difficult to calculate D' by hand, but a number of computer programs are available (e.g. Centor and Schwartz 1985; Dorfman and Alf 1969). The standard error of the ROC is given by Hanley and McNeil (1982) as:

$$SE = \left[\frac{D'(1 - D') + (N_c - 1) Q_1 - D'^2) + (N_n - 1) (Q_2 - D'^2)}{N_c N_n} \right]^{\frac{1}{2}}$$

where $Q_1 = D'/(2 - D')$,

$Q_2 = 2 D'2 / (1 - D')$,

N_c = number of cases, and

N_n = number of non-cases.

We mentioned previously that the cut point nearest the upper left corner resulted in the smallest overall error rate. There may be some circumstances,

Table 7.6   *Calculations for an ROC curve*

Cut-Off	Case	Non-case	Cut-Off	Case	Non-case	Cut-Off	Case	Non-case
10	49	0	11	136	5	10–12	228	9
11–20	441	500	12–20	364	495	13–20	272	491

Cut Point	True Positives	False Positives	Sensitivity	1 – Specificity
< 10	0	0	0.000	0.000
10	49	0	0.098	0.000
11	136	5	0.272	0.010
12	228	9	0.456	0.018
13	311	18	0.622	0.036
14	369	48	0.738	0.096
15	437	118	0.874	0.236
16	466	179	0.932	0.358
17	491	235	0.982	0.470
18	495	361	0.990	0.722
19	500	474	1.000	0.948
20	500	500	1.000	1.000

though, where it may be preferable to move this point, either up or down, even though the number of false positives or false negatives may increase faster than the number of true positives. For example, if the consequences of missing a case can be tragic, and second-level tests exist which can weed out the false positives (as with HIV sero-conversion), then the cut-off point may be lowered. Conversely, if there are more good applicants than positions, as is the case in admission requests for graduate or professional school, then it makes sense to raise the cut-off. The cost will be an increased number of false negatives (i.e. potentially good students who are denied admission), but relatively few false positives.

Age and sex norms

Some attributes, especially those assessed in adults like cardiac output, show relatively little change with age and do not differ between males and females. Other factors, such as measures of lung capacity like FVC, show considerable

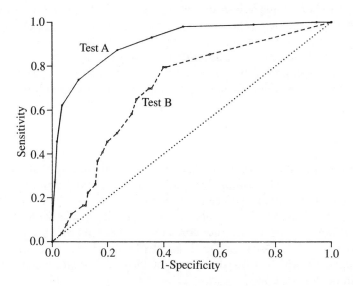

Fig. 7.3. Example of an ROC curve.

variation with age or gender. It is well known, for example, that females are more prone to admit to depressive symptomatology than are men. The psychometric solution to this problem is relatively easy: separate norms can be developed for each sex, as was done for the Depression scale and some others on the MMPI. However, this may mask a more important and fundamental difficulty; do the sexes differ only in terms of their willingness to endorse depressive items, or does this reflect more actual depression in women? Separate norms assume that the distribution of depression is equivalent for males and females, and it is only the reporting that is different.

The opposite approach was taken by Wechsler (1958) in constructing his intelligence tests. He began with the explicit assumption that males and females do not differ on any of the dimensions that his instruments tap. During the process of developing the tests, he therefore discarded any tasks, such as spatial relations, which did show a systematic bias between the sexes.

These decisions were *theoretically founded* ones, not psychometric ones, based on the developer's conception of how these attributes exist in reality. Deciding whether sex norms should be used (as with the MMPI) or whether more endorsed items means more underlying depression (as in the Beck or Zung scales), or if the sexes *should* differ on some trait such as intelligence reflects a theoretical model. Since these are crucial in interpreting the results, they should be spelled out explicitly in any manual or paper about the instrument.

Age norms are less contentious, as developmental changes are more objective and verifiable. Some of the many examples of age-related differences are height, weight, or vocabulary. When these exist, separate norms are developed for each age group, and often age-sex group, as boys and girls develop at different rates. The major question facing the test constructor is how large the age span should be in each normative group. The answer depends to a large degree on the speed of maturation of the trait; a child should not change in his or her percentile level too much in crossing from the upper limit of one age group to the beginning of the next. If this does occur, then it is probable that the age span is too great.

Summary

We have covered three points in this chapter. First, differential weighting of items rarely is worth the trouble. Second, if a test is being developed for local use only, it would probably suffice to use simply the sum of the items. However, for more general use, and to be able to compare the results with other instruments, it is better to transform the scores into percentiles, and best to transform them into z-scores or T-scores. Third, for attributes which differ between males and females, or which show development changes, separate age or age-sex norms can be developed.

References

Beck, A. T., Ward, C. H., Mendelson, M., Mock, J., and Erbaugh, J. (1961). An inventory for measuring depression. *Archives of General Psychiatry*, **4**, 561–71.

Cattell, R. B., Eber, H. W., and Tatsuoka, M. M. (1970). *Handbook for the Sixteen Personality Factor Questionnaire (16PF)*. Institute for Personality and Ability Testing, Champaign, IL.

Centor, R. M. and Schwartz, J. S. (1985). An evaluation of methods for estimating the error under the receiver operating characteristic (ROC) curve. *Medical Decision Making*, **5**, 149–56.

Dorfman, D. D. and Alf, E. (1969). Maximum likelihood estimation of parameters of signal detection theory and determination of confidence intervals-rating-method data. *Journal of Mathematical Psychology*, **6**, 487–96.

Evans, M. G. (1991). The problem of analyzing multiplicative composites: Interactions revisited. *American Psychologist*, **46**, 6–15.

Gulliksen, H. O. (1950). *Theory of mental tests*. Wiley, New York.

Hanley, J. A. and McNeil, B. J. (1982). The meaning and use of the area under a receiver operating characteristics (ROC) curve. *Radiology*, **143**, 29–36.

Holmes, T. H. and Rahe, R. H. (1967). The social readjustment rating scale. *Journal of Psychosomatic Research*, **11**, 213–18.

Jackson, D. N. (1984). *Personality Research Form manual*. Research Psychologists Press, Port Huron, MI.

Jenkinson, C. (1991). Why are we weighting? A critical examination of the use of item weights in a health status measure. *Social Science and Medicine*, **32**, 1413–16.

Lei, H. and Skinner, H. A. (1980). A psychometric study of life events and social readjustment. *Journal of Psychosomatic Research*, **24**, 57–65.

Norman, G. R. and Streiner, D. L. (1994). *Biostatistics: The bare essentials*. Mosby, St Louis, MO.

Nunnally, J. C., Jr. (1970). *Introduction to psychological measurement*. McGraw-Hill, New York.

Perloff, J. M. and Persons, J. B. (1988). Biases resulting from the use of indexes: An application to attributional style and depression. *Psychological Bulletin*, **103**, 95–104.

Peterson, W. W., Birdshall, T. G., and Fox, W. C. (1954). The theory of signal detectability. *IRE Transactions: Professional Group on Information Theory*, **4**, 171–212.

Retzlaff, P. D., Sheehan, E. P., and Lorr, M. (1990). MCMI-II scoring: Weighted and unweighted algorithms. *Journal of Personality Assessment*, **55**, 219–23.

Streiner, D. L., Goldberg, J. O., and Miller, H. R. (1993). MCMI-II weights: Their lack of effectiveness. *Journal of Personality Assessment*, **60**, 471–6.

Streiner, D. L. and Miller, H. R. (1989). The MCMI-II: How much better than the MCMI? *Journal of Personality Assessment*, **53**, 81–4.

Streiner, D. L., Norman, G. R., McFarlane, A. H., and Roy, R. G. (1981). Quality of life events and their relationship to strain. *Schizophrenia Bulletin*, **7**, 34–42.

Tanner, W. P., Jr. and Swets, J. A. (1954). A decision making theory of visual detection. *Psychological Review*, **61**, 401–9.

Wainer, H. (1976). Estimating coefficients in linear models: It don't make no nevermind. *Psychological Bulletin*, **83**, 213–17.

Wechsler, D. (1958). *The measurement and appraisal of adult human intelligence* (4th edn.). Williams and Wilkins, Baltimore.

Wechsler, D. (1981). *WAIS-R manual: Wechsler Adult Intelligence Scale-Revised*. Psychological Corporation, New York.

Zung, W. K. (1965). A self-rating depression scale. *Archives of General Psychiatry*, **12**, 63–70.

8

Reliability

The concept of *reliability* is a fundamental way to reflect the amount of error, both random and systematic, inherent in any measurement. Yet despite its essential role in judgements of the adequacy of any measurement process, it is devilishly difficult to achieve a real understanding of the psychometric approach to reliability. Some health science researchers also tend to cloud the issue by invoking a long list of possible synonyms, such as 'objectivity', 'reproducibility', 'stability', 'agreement', 'association', 'sensitivity', and 'precision'. Since few of these terms have a formal definition, we will not attempt to show how each differs from the other. Instead, we will concern ourselves with a detailed explanation of the concept of reliability. While some of the terms will be singled out for special treatment later in the chapter, primarily to emphasize their shortcomings, others will be ignored.

Our reasons for this apparently single-minded viewpoint are simple. The technology of reliability assessment was worked out very early in the history of psychological assessment. We once traced its roots back to a textbook written in the 1930s, and the basic definitions were given without reference, indicating that, even six decades ago, the classical definition was viewed as uncontroversial. There is complete consensus within the educational and psychological communities regarding the meaning of the term, and disagreement and debate are confined to a small cadre of biomedical researchers. Moreover, once one understands the basic concept it appears, in our view, to reflect perfectly the particular requirements of any measurement situation. Although there are some more recent theories in education and psychology, such as generalizability theory (see Chapter 9), these represent extensions of the basic approach. Other conflicting views which have arisen in the biomedical research community, such as the treatment of Bland and Altman (1986) are, in our view, fundamentally flawed. This latter method, because of its recent popularity, will be discussed separately.

Basic concepts

What is this elusive concept, and why is it apparently so hard to understand? In order to explore it, we will begin with some commonsense notions of measurement error, and eventually link them to the more formal definitions of reliability.

Daily experience constantly reminds us of measurement error. We leap or crawl out of bed in the morning, and step on the scales. We know to disregard any changes less than about 2 lb or 1 kg, since bathroom scales are typically accurate to no better than ±2 lb (±1 kg). If our children are ill, we may measure their temperature with a home thermometer, accurate to about ±0.2°C. Baby's weight gain or loss is measured on a different scale, at home or at the doctor's surgery, accurate to about ±20 gm. As we eat breakfast, we note the time on the wall, and implicitly recognize that if the clock has hands, there is a likely measurement error of about 5 minutes; if it displays numbers, the error is probably a fraction of a minute. Before donning our coat to leave the house, we check the outside thermometer (±2°F, ±1C). We leap into our cars and accelerate rapidly up to the speed limit, at least as assessed by our car's speedometer (±5 km/hr; ±3 mph), and check the time again as we arrive at work, by looking at our wristwatches (they're probably quartz, ±15 sec). We settle at our desks, pick up the first cup of coffee or tea of the day, and read a new paper on observer error which begins by stating that 'the reliability was calculated with an intraclass correlation, and equalled 0.86'.

Why, for goodness sake, do we have to create some arcane statistic, with no dimension and a range from zero to one, regardless of the measurement situation, in order to express measurement error? To explain, let us review the measurements of the previous paragraph. We begin by assuming that the reader will accept that the measurement errors we cited, while not precisely correct, were at least approximately consistent with our common experience. In the brief 'Day in the Life of...', we indicated two measurements of time, weight, and temperature, each with an approximate error. We are completely comfortable with a bathroom scale accurate to ±1 kg, since we know that individual weights vary over far greater ranges than this, and typical changes from day to day are about the same order of magnitude. Conversely, we recognize that this error of measurement is unacceptable for weighing infants, because it exceeds important changes in weight. Similarly, an error of time measurement of several minutes is usually small compared with the anticipated tolerances in daily life (except for European trains). Indeed, many people have now reverted back to quartz analog watches, since they find the extreme accuracy of the digital readouts unnecessary and annoying. Finally, we tolerate an error of measurement of several degrees Celsius for outside air temperature, since we know that it may range from −40° to +60° Celsius (in the UK, from −5 to +15), so the measurement error is a small fraction of the true range. The same measurement error is, however, hopeless in a clinical situation since body temperature is restricted to a range of only a few degrees.

In all of these situations, our comfort resides in the knowledge that the error of measurement is a relatively small fraction of the range in the observations. Further, the reason that the measurement error alone provides useful information in the everyday world is that we share a common perception of the expected differences we will encounter. However, such everyday information is conspicuously absent for many measurement scales. To report that the error of measurement on a new depression scale is ±3 is of little value since we do not know the degree of difference among patients, or between patients and non-patients. In order to provide useful information about measurement error, it must be contrasted with the expected variation amongst the individuals we may be assessing.

One way to include the information about expected variability between patients would be to cite the ratio of measurement error to total variability between patients. Since the total variability between patients includes both any systematic variation between patients and measurement error, this would result in a number between zero and one, with zero representing a 'perfect' instrument. Such a ratio would then indicate the ability of the instrument to differentiate among patients. In practice, the ratio is turned around, and researchers calculate the ratio of variability *between* patients to the *total* variability (the sum of patient variability and measurement error), so that zero indicates no reliability, and one indicates no measurement error and perfect reliability. Thus the formal definition of reliability is:

$$Reliability = \frac{Subject\ Variability}{Subject\ Variability\ +\ Measurement\ Error}$$

Since one statistical measure of variability is *variance*, this can be expressed more formally as:

$$Reliability = \frac{\sigma^2_s}{\sigma^2_s + \sigma^2_e}$$

where the '*s*' subscript stands for 'Subjects', and the '*e*' for Error.

Thus the reliability coefficient expresses the proportion of the total variance in the measurements ($\sigma^2_s + \sigma^2_e$) which is due to 'true' differences between subjects (σ^2_s). As we shall see, 'true' is defined in a very particular way, but this awaits a detailed discussion of the methods of calculation.

Philosophical implications

This formulation of reliability has profound consequences for the logic of measurement. At its root, the reliability coefficient reflects the extent to which a measurement instrument can differentiate among individuals, i.e. how well it can tell people apart, since the magnitude of the coefficient is directly related to the variability between subjects. The concept seems restrictively Darwinian and even feudal. But this interpretation is a political not a scientific one, and perhaps reflects a focus on the potentially negative use to which the measurement may be put, rather than the measurement itself.

Reflect back again on the everyday use of measurement. The only reason to apply a particular instrument to a situation is because the act of measurement is providing information about the object of observation. We look at the thermometer outside only because it tells us something about how this day differs from all other days. If the thermometer always gave the same reading because every day was the same temperature as every other day, we would soon stop reading it. We suspect, although we lack direct experience, that because of this people living in tropical climates pay little attention to the temperature, and that other factors, such as rain or humidity, are more important.

This intuition applies equally well to clinical and other professional situations. A laboratory measurement is useful only to the extent that it reflects true differences among individuals; in particular diseased and normal individuals. Chromosome count is not a useful genetic property (despite the fact that we can get perfect agreement among observers) because we all have 46 chromosomes. Similarly, most clinical supervisors question the value of global rating scales (the bit of paper routinely filled out by the supervisor at the end of an educational experience rating everything from knowledge to responsibility) precisely because everybody, from the best to the worst, gets rated 'above average'.

Again, this view flies in the face of some further intuitions. Reliability is not necessarily related to agreement, and in some cases can be inversely related to it. We have just demonstrated one example, where if all students on all occasions are rated above average, the agreement among raters is perfect but the reliability, by definition, is zero. This is also relevant to the 'number of boxes' issue discussed in Chapter 4. As we decrease the number of boxes on a rating scale, the information value of any observation is reduced, and the reliability drops, although the agreement among observers will increase. As an everyday example, Canadians now uniformly talk about the weather in degrees Celsius, but still refer to room temperature in degrees Fahrenheit. We think one reason for this phenomenon is that within the range of acceptable room temperature, from say 68° to 72° Fahrenheit or 20° to 21° Celsius (except the United Kingdom where the lower limit, particularly in bathrooms, is more like 32°F or 0°C), the Celsius scale has only two divisions compared to four for the Fahrenheit one, thus introducing a degree of measurement error, even though two thermometers would agree (within one degree) more often in Celsius.

Experimentalists, and many statisticians, have difficulty with the concept of reliability as well. To the experimentalist, the goal of science is to detect the effects of experimental interventions. This 'main effect', in a comparison between treatment and control groups, for example, is always confounded, to greater or lesser degree, by differences in individual subjects' responses. Nearly all statistical tests make this contrast explicit; the numerator of the test is the experimental effect, assessed as differences between means, differences in proportions cured or dead, and so on, and the denominator is the expected magnitude of the difference by chance *arising from differences among individuals*. Thus, it is precisely true that the psychometrician's (and arguably, the clinician's) *signal* is the experimentalist's and statistician's *noise*.

This paradox was first recognized by Cronbach, the inventor of the alpha coefficient (Chapter 5) and generalizability theory (Chapter 9), in a classic paper written in 1957, called "The two disciplines of scientific psychology". Perhaps because of the title, few readers outside psychology (and regrettably, few inside as well) are aware of it. The paradox rears its ugly head in many areas of research.

As one example, clinical researchers often go to great lengths to create inclusion and exclusion criteria in order to enrol just the right kind of (homogeneous) patients in their studies. Sometimes they go to extreme lengths, such as one trial of a cholesterol lowering drug which screened 300 000 men in order to find 4000 who fit the criteria. It is often forgotten that the reason for these extreme measures is because the small treatment effects common in cardiovascular research would be obscured by individual differences if all kinds of patients were enrolled.

On the analysis side, although we use standard statistical packages to develop reliability coefficients, it is literally true that every line in the ANOVA table of concern in these calculations is labelled 'ERROR' by most of the standard packages. Conversely, the 'main effects', or differences between means, which are of interest to the statisticians are frequently (but not always) ignored in the calculations of reliability.

There is one last important consequence of this formulation. The reliability of a measure is intimately linked to the population to which one wants to apply the measure. There is literally no such thing as the reliability of a test, unqualified; the coefficient has meaning only when applied to specific populations. Reliability is relative, just as Einstein said about time. Although some researchers (Bland and Altman 1986) have decried this as a failure of conventional methods for assessing reliability, we believe that this is a realistic view of the act of measurement, and not a limitation of reliability. Returning to the introduction, it makes no sense to speak of the error of measurement of a thermometer without knowledge of the range of temperature to be assessed. Small differences amongst the objects of measurement are more difficult to detect than large differences. The reliability coefficient explicitly recognizes this important characteristic.

Defining the reliability of a test

So far, we have described the idea of reliability in general terms. The time has come to define how to calculate reliability; that is, how to determine the different variance components which enter into the coefficient. Perhaps not surprisingly, the analytical approach is based on the statistical technique of Analysis of Variance (ANOVA). Specifically, because we have repeated observations on each subject or patient derived from different observers, times, or versions of the test, we use a method called repeated measures ANOVA.

Table 8.1 *Degree of sadness on 10 patients rated by 3 observers*

Patient	Observer 1	Observer 2	Observer 3	Mean
1	6	7	8	7.0
2	4	5	6	5.0
3	2	2	2	2.0
4	3	4	5	4.0
5	5	4	6	5.0
6	8	9	10	9.0
7	5	7	9	7.0
8	6	7	8	7.0
9	4	6	8	6.0
10	7	9	8	8.0
Mean	5.0	6.0	7.0	6.00

Suppose, for example, that three observers assess a total of 10 patients for some attribute (e.g. sadness) on a 10-point scale. The scores are shown in Table 8.1.

It is evident that there is some variability in the scores. Those assigned by the three observers to individual patients range from 2 to 10 units on the scale, with mean scores ranging from 2 to 9. The variability among the mean scores of the observers (5.0 *vs.* 6.0 *vs.* 7.0) suggests that there may be some systematic difference among them. Finally, there is as much as two units of disagreement in scores assigned to the same patient by different observers.

These three sources of variance—patients, observers, and error—are represented in different ways in the table: the patients, by the differences within the column on the right (their means); the observers, by the differences among their three column means; and 'random', or unsystematic variation, by the difference between an individual score within the table and its 'expected' value. Thus we have adopted a technical estimate of the 'true' score; it is simply the average of all the observed scores, whether applied to the true score of a patient (i.e. each patient's mean) or of an observer (their means). 'True' clearly has a technical definition which is somewhat more limited than the common definition. In particular, it does not mean that the average of the scores in any way represents the true value of the underlying characteristic (in this case, sadness) being assessed; that is a job for validity assessment. In any case, these sources of variance are initially quantified in sums of squares, calculated as below:

$$\text{Sum of squares (observers)} = 10[(5.0 - 6.0)^2 + (6.0 - 6.0)^2 + (7.0 - 6.0)^2] = 20.0.$$

Table 8.2 *Analysis of variance summary table*

Source of variation	Sum of squares	Degrees of freedom	Mean square	F	Tail probability
Patients	114.00	9	12.67	22.80	0.0001
Raters	20.00	2	10.00	18.00	0.0001
Error	10.00	18	0.56		
Total	144.00	29			

The factor of 10 is there because 10 patients enter into each sum. Similarly:

$$\text{Sum of squares (patients)} = 3[(7.0 - 6.0)^2 + (5.0 - 6.0)^2 + (2.0 - 6.0^2 + \ldots + (8.0 - 6.0)^2] = 114.0$$

Again, there is a factor of 3 in the equation because there are three observers contributing to each value.

Finally, the sum of squares (Error) is based on the difference between each individual value and its expected value calculated from the row and column means. We will not go into detail about how these expected values are arrived at; any introductory text book in statistics, such as Norman and Streiner (1994), will explain it. For the first three patients and Observer 1, the expected scores are 6.0, 5.5, and 4.5. The sum of squares is then:

$$\text{Sum of squares (error)} = (6.0 - 6.0)^2 + (5.0 - 5.5)^2 + (4.0 - 4.5)^2 + \ldots + (8.0 - 9.0)^2 = 10.0.$$

An ANOVA table can then be developed from the sums of squares, as in Table 8.2.

The next step is to break down the total variance in the scores into components of variance due to patients, observers, and error. It would seem that each mean square is a variance, and no further work is required, but such is not the case. Both the calculated mean square due to patients and that due to observers contain some contribution due to error variance. The easiest way to understand this concept is to imagine a situation where all patients had the same degree of sadness, as defined by some external gold standard. Would the patients all then obtain the same scores on our sadness scale? Not at all. There would be variability in the obtained scores directly related to the amount of random error present in the measurements. The relevant equations relating the mean square (MSs) to variances are below:

- Mean square (error) $= \sigma^2_{\text{Err}}$
- Mean square (patients) $= 3\sigma^2_{\text{Pat}} + \sigma^2_{\text{Err}}$
- Mean square (observers) $= 10\sigma^2_{\text{Obs}} + \sigma^2_{\text{Err}}$

From these we can show, by some algebraic manipulations, that:

- $\sigma^2(\text{error}) = MS_{Err} = 0.56$
- $\sigma^2(\text{patients}) = (MS_{Pat} - MS_{Err})/3 = (12.67 - 0.56)/3 = 4.04$
- $\sigma^2(\text{observers}) = (MS_{Obs} - MS_{Err})/10 = (10.00 - 0.56)/10 = 0.94$

Finally, we are in a position to define the reliability coefficient as the ratio of variance between patients to error variance.

$$R = \frac{\sigma^2_{patients}}{\sigma^2_{patients} + \sigma^2_{error}} = \frac{4.04}{4.04 + 0.56} = 0.88$$

This is the 'classical' definition of reliability. The interpretation is that 88 per cent of the variance in the scores results from 'true' variance among patients. The coefficient is called an *Intraclass correlation coefficient* or ICC. (Note first that it is not *the* ICC; as we shall see, there are different forms of it, depending on various assumptions we make. Also note that it is the reliability coefficient, r, and not r^2, which is interpreted as the percentage of score variance attributable to different sources.)

Other considerations in calculating the reliability of a test

The observation as a fixed or random factor

What happened to the variance due to observer? Although it was calculated in the ANOVA table, and was found to be highly significant, there was no further mention of it. Conventional treatments of reliability consistently omit the main effect associated with observations, and we have found only one reference (Shrout and Fleiss 1979) which deals explicitly with this issue.

Whether Observer should or should not be included is a decision which is dependent on whether we wish to treat observations as a fixed or random factor. For example, if the eventual application of the test will always use the same observers who were involved in the reliability study, then the observers have been 'calibrated'. Any score obtained from the first observer should have 1.0 added, and one from the third observer should have 1.0 subtracted. If such a correction factor is applied, then there is no reason to include this observer bias in the reliability coefficient. In fact, if all the subsequent patients will always be assessed by all of the same three observers, we need not apply any correction, since the plus and minus ones will always be present.

Other situations where the observation might be treated as a fixed factor occur when the observations arise from various items on a scale, such as 'I feel tired most of the time' on a depression scale or different questions on a short answer test. This form of reliability is known as *internal consistency* and was first encountered in Chapter 5; we will treat it more fully below. Since all participants complete the same items, we can safely treat the observation (i.e. the item) as a fixed factor. Historically, since much of psychometric theory was worked out on aptitude or personality tests of this form, we believe that this led to the convention of omitting the main effect of observation from the coefficient.

Conversely, if the observers in the reliability study are intended to be a random sample of a number of possible observers, or if no correction can be applied, then observer bias can result in a further error introduced into any individual score. In this case, the bias should be included in the reliability coefficient. The resulting coefficient would look like:

$$R = \frac{\sigma^2_{subjects}}{\sigma^2_{subjects} + \sigma^2_{observers} + \sigma^2_{error}} = \frac{4.04}{4.04 + 0.56 + 0.94} = 0.73$$

which is a different variant of the ICC.

The observer nested within subject

One common situation arises when each subject is rated by several different observers, but no observers are common to more than one subject. Some examples would be: students in a course in different tutorial groups rate their tutors' teaching skills; junior residents on different teaching units are rated by chief residents, head nurses, and staff; and patients undergoing physiotherapy are rated by their own and another therapist, but treatment is given by different therapists at different hospitals. Common to these situations is that (a) all subjects receive more than one observation, but (b) no observer rates more than one subject.

At first glance, it would seem impossible to extract a reliability coefficient from these data, since there seems to be no opportunity to actually compare observations. Certainly in the extreme case, where each subject is rated by only one observer, there is no way to separate subject variance, observer variance, and error. But in the situations above, at least a partial separation can be achieved.

The approach is to recognize that the variance of the mean values of the scores of each subject permits an estimate of subject variance, in the usual way. Conversely, variability of the observations around the mean of each subject is a result of within-subject variation, contributed by both systematic differences between observers and error variance. We cannot separate these two sources of variance but we do not really need to, since the denominator of the reliability coefficient contains contributions from both.

To analyse data of this form, we conduct a one-way ANOVA with the subject as a grouping factor, and the multiple observations within each subject cell as a 'within-subject' factor. We need not have the same number of observers for each subject, as long as the number of observations per subject exceeds one.

The one-way ANOVA results, eventually, in estimated mean squares between groups and within groups. The former is used to calculate subject variance, using the previous formula, and the mean square (within) estimates the error variance. The reliability coefficient can then be calculated with these variance estimates, using the conventional formula. All that is lost is the ability to separate the random error component from observer bias; but since observers are a random effect (using the concepts described in the previous subsection), this is of no consequence.

Even in those situations where there is partial overlap (for example, 15 interview teams of three interviewers conduct 10 interviews each), the analysis can be approached assuming no overlap of raters, and still yield an unbiased estimate of reliability.

Multiple observations

Finally, let us re-examine the issue of multiple observations. If each patient is assessed by multiple observers, or completes some inventory with a number of items, or fills out a pain scale on several occasions, it is intuitively obvious that the average of these observations should have a higher reliability than any single item, since the errors are random, and those associated with each observation are averaged out. In turn, this should be reflected in the reliability coefficient.

The approach is the essence of simplicity: we simply divide the error variance by the number of observations. So, if all three observers were involved and their scores were averaged, the reliability of this average score is:

$$R = \frac{4.04}{4.04 + \dfrac{(0.56 + 0.94)}{3}} = 0.89$$

Similarly, for a multi-item inventory, we would omit the main effect of item (observation) and divide the error term by the number of items, k:

$$\text{Reliability (k items)} = \frac{\sigma^2_{Subject}}{\sigma^2_{Subject} + \dfrac{\sigma^2_{Error}}{k}}$$

This is the original form of the alpha coefficient. The formula in Chapter 5 arises from simplifications based on the actual computations.

Other types of reliability

Up to this point, we have concerned ourselves with reliability as a measure of association, examining the effect of different observers on scores. The example we have worked through included only one source of error, that which resulted from different observers' perceptions of the same behaviour. Upon reflection, we can see that there may be other sources of error or contamination in an observation of an individual patient's 'sadness'. For instance, each observer may apply slightly different standards from day to day. This could be tested experimentally by videotaping a group of patients and having the observer do two ratings of the tapes a week or two apart. The resulting reliability is called an *intra-observer reliability* coefficient, since it measures variation which occurs within an observer as a result of multiple exposures to the same stimulus, as opposed to the *inter-observer* reliability we have already calculated.

Note that although many investigators maintain that the demonstration of both inter- and intra-observer reliability is a minimum requirement of a good test, this may be unnecessary. If we recognize that inter-observer reliability contains all the sources of error contributing to intra-observer reliability, plus any differences which may arise between observers, then it is evident that a demonstration of high inter-observer reliability is sufficient; the intra-observer reliability is bound to be higher. However, if the inter-observer reliability is low, we cannot be sure whether this arises from differences within or between observers (or both), and it may then be necessary to continue to an intra-observer reliability study in order to locate the source of unreliability.

Often there are no observers involved in the measurement, as with the many self-rated tests of psychological function, pain, or disease severity. Although there are no observers, we are still concerned about the reliability of the scale. The usual approach is to administer it on two occasions separated by a time interval sufficiently short that we can assume that the underlying process is unlikely to have changed. This approach is called *test–retest reliability*. Of course, the trick is to select an appropriate time interval: too long, and things may have changed; too short, and patients may remember their first response and put it down, rather than answering the question *de novo*. Expert opinions regarding the appropriate interval vary from an hour to a year depending on the task, but generally speaking, a retest interval of two to 14 days is usual. (The section on *Empirical data on retest reliability*, later in this chapter, shows the magnitude of the coefficient expected for various types of tests after different intervals.)

Frequently, measures of internal consistency, as described in Chapter 5, are reported as the reliability of a test. However, since they are based on performance observed in a single sitting, there are many sources of variance which occur from day to day or between observers which do not enter into the calculation. Because they can be computed from routine administration of a measure, without the special requirement for two or more administrations, they appear very commonly in the literature but should be interpreted with great caution.

Different forms of the reliability coefficient

There has been considerable debate in the literature regarding the most appropriate choice of the reliability coefficient. The coefficients we have derived to now are all forms of 'intraclass correlation coefficients'. However, other

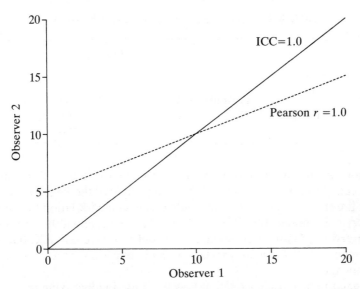

Fig. 8.1. Typical graph of inter-observer scores, showing difference between Pearson correlation and intraclass correlation.

measures, in particular the Pearson product-moment correlation and Cohen's kappa (Cohen 1960), are frequently used. Altman and Bland (1983; Bland and Altman 1986) have also identified apparent weaknesses in the conventional approach and recommended an alternative. Accordingly, we will discuss these alternatives, and attempt to reconcile the differences among the measures.

Pearson correlation

The Pearson correlation is based on regression analysis, and is a measure of the extent to which the relationship between two variables can be described by a straight (regression) line. In the present context, this is a measure of the extent to which two observations on a group of subjects can be fitted by a straight line. One such relationship is shown in Figure 8.1. Note that a perfect fit is obtained, resulting in a Pearson correlation of 1.0, despite the fact that the intercept is non-zero and the slope is not equal to 1.0. By contrast, the intraclass correlation will yield a value of 1.0 only if all the observations on each subject are identical, which dictates a slope of 1.0 and an intercept of 0.0. This suggests that the Pearson correlation is an inappropriate and liberal measure of reliability; that is to say, the Pearson coefficient will usually be higher than the true reliability. In practice, however, the predominant source of error is usually due to random variation, and under these circumstances, the Pearson and intraclass correlations will be very close.

There is a second reason to prefer the intraclass correlation over the Pearson

Table 8.3   *Contingency Table for two observers*

		Observer 2		
		Present	Absent	Total
	Present	20	15	35
Observer 1	Absent	10	55	65
	Total	30	70	100

correlation. We began this chapter with an example which used three observers, and proceeded to calculate a single ICC. If we had used the Pearson correlation, we must use the data pairwise, and would create one correlation for Observer 1 *vs*. Observer 2, another for Observer 1 *vs*. Observer 3, and a third for Observer 2 *vs*. Observer 3. With 10 observers, we would still have one ICC but we must now contend with 45 Pearson correlations, and there is no agreed way to average or combine them.

Although the pairwise correlation may be of use in identifying particular outlier examiners for further training, in general we presume that the observers are a random sample of all possible observers, and we have no particular interest in individuals. In these circumstances, it is of considerable value to use all the data to estimate a single ICC representing the average correlation between any two observers.

Kappa coefficient

Although this chapter (and most of this book) has dealt at length with situations where there is a supposed underlying continuum, there are many situations in medicine which have only two levels—presence or absence, positive or negative, abnormal or normal, dead or alive (although with cardiac and electroencephalic monitoring, disagreement is rare in the latter instance). A straightforward approach is to calculate simple agreement: the proportion of responses in which the two observations agreed. Although straightforward, this measure is very strongly influenced by the distribution of positives and negatives. If there is a preponderance of either normal or abnormal cases, there will be a high agreement by chance alone. The kappa coefficient (Cohen 1960) explicitly deals with this situation by examining the proportion of responses in the two agreement cells (yes/yes, no/no) in relation to the proportion of responses in these cells which would be expected by chance, given the marginal distributions.

For example, suppose we were to consider a judgement by two observers of the presence or absence of a Babinski sign (an upgoing toe following scratching of the bottom of the foot) on a series of neurological patients. The data might be displayed in a contingency table like Table 8.3.

The overall agreement is simply (20 + 55)/100 = 75%. However, we would expect that a certain number of agreements would arise by chance alone. Specifically, we can calculate the expected agreement from the marginals; the top left cell would have $(35 \times 30)/100 = 10.5$ expected observations, and the bottom right cell would have $(70 \times 65)/100 = 45.5$ expected ones. Kappa corrects for chance agreement in the following manner:

$$\varkappa = \frac{P_o - P_e}{1.0 - P_e}$$

where P_o is the observed proportion of agreements, and P_e is the proportion expected by chance. In this case:

$$\varkappa = \frac{\left(\dfrac{75}{100}\right) - \left(\dfrac{10.5 + 45.5}{100}\right)}{1.0 - \left(\dfrac{10.5 + 45.5}{100}\right)} = 0.43$$

For a 2 × 2 table, we can also calculate the standard error of the kappa:

$$SE\,(\varkappa) = \sqrt{\frac{P_o(1 - P_o)}{N(1.0 - P_e)^2}}$$

which in this case equals:

$$\sqrt{\frac{0.75\,(1 - 0.75)}{100\,(1.0 - 0.56)^2}} = 0.098$$

Therefore, instead of a raw agreement of 0.75, we end up with a chance-corrected agreement of 0.43, with a standard error of about 0.10. In circumstances where the frequency of positive results is very low or very high, it is very easy to obtain impressive figures for agreement although agreement beyond chance is virtually absent.

In the example we have chosen, the approach to assessment of observer agreement appears to have little in common with our previous examples, where we used ANOVA methods. However, if we considered judgements which differ only slightly from Babinski signs, the parallel may become more obvious. For example, suppose the same observers were assessing muscle strength, which is conventionally done on a 6-point scale from 0=flaccid to 5=normal strength. In this case, a display of agreement would involve a 6 × 6 contingency table.

Since the coefficient we calculated previously considers only total agreement and does not provide partial credit for responses which differ by only one or two categories, it would be inappropriate for scaled responses as in the present example. However, an extension of the approach, called *weighted kappa* (Cohen 1968), does consider partial agreement.

Weighted kappa actually focuses on disagreement, so that the cells of total agreement on the top left to bottom right diagonal have weights of zero and two opposite corners have the maximum weights. Weighted kappa is then a sum of the weighted frequencies corrected for chance. The actual formula is:

$$\varkappa_w = 1.0 - \frac{\sum w_{ij} \times P_{o_{ij}}}{\sum w_{ij} \times P_{e_{ij}}}$$

where w is the weight assigned to the i,j cell, and p_{oij} and p_{eij} are the observed and expected proportions in the i,j cell.

As originally formulated, the weights could be assigned arbitrary values between 0 and 1. However, the problem with using your own weights, however sensible they may seem, is that you can no longer compare your kappa with anyone else's. Unless there are strong prior reasons the most commonly used weighting scheme, called *quadratic weights*, which bases disagreement weights on the square of the amount of discrepancy, should be used. *If this weighting scheme is used, then the weighted kappa is exactly identical to the intraclass correlation coefficient* (Fleiss and Cohen 1973). If numbers are assigned to each cell (in the case of our second example, from one to six) and then analysed using ANOVA methods, the resulting intraclass correlation will be identical to the unweighted kappa. Similarly, if the two cells in the original table are assigned the numbers 0 and 1 (or, for that matter, any numbers), the unweighted kappa is also equal to an ICC based on analysis of variance. Needless to say, this observation makes things a lot simpler.

The method of Bland and Altman

An alternative method of examining agreement was proposed by Altman and Bland (1983; Bland and Altman 1986), which has the apparent virtue of independence of the true variability in the observations. We have discussed earlier in this chapter why we would view this independence as a liability, not an asset. However, because this method has achieved considerable prominence in the British clinical literature, we will review it in detail.

The method is designed as an absolute measure of agreement between two measuring instruments which are on the same scale of measurement. As such, it retains the virtue of the intraclass correlation, in contrast to the Pearson correlation, in explicitly separating the bias (or main) effect of the instrument from random error. The approach is used for pairs of observations, and begins with a plot of the difference between the two observations against the mean of the pairs of observations. One then calculates the average difference in the observations, and the standard deviation of the differences. The mean difference is analytically related to the observer variance calculated in the ICC (actually, it equals $\sqrt{(2/n)} \cdot MS_{osb}$. The standard deviation of the differences is similarly related to the error variance ($\sqrt{MS_{err}}$). A statistical test of the observer bias can be performed, and would yield the same significance level as the test in the ANOVA. Finally, one calculates the *limits of agreement*, equal to the mean difference ± twice the standard error.

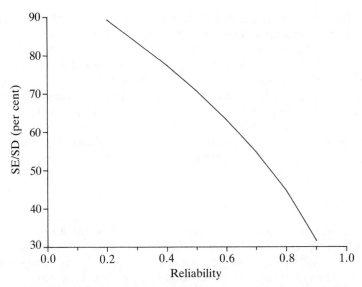

Fig. 8.2. Relation between reliability and standard error of measurement.

Agreement is therefore expressed by the 'limit of agreement', which is analytically related to the error variance in our previous calculation. As we have already indicated, while the method has advantages over the Pearson correlation in the explicit dissociation between systematic and random error, this advantage is shared by the ICC. The apparent advantage of creating a coefficient which is independent of the true variation in the sample of observations is, in our view, illusory, and places on the reader the onus to juxtapose the calculated error against some implicit notion of true variability.

Issues of interpretation

Reliability and the standard error of measurement

One difficulty with expressing the reliability coefficient as a dimensionless ratio of variances instead of an error of measurement is that it is difficult to interpret a reliability coefficient of 0.7 in terms of an individual score. However, since the reliability coefficient involves two quantities—the error variance and the variance between subjects—it is straightforward to work backwards and express the error of measurement in terms of the other two quantities. The *standard error of measurement (SEM)* is defined in terms of the standard deviation (σ) and the reliability (R) as:

$$SEM = \sigma \sqrt{1 - R}$$

This relationship is plotted for some values of reliability in Figure 8.2. The interpretation of this graph is that if we begin with a sample of known standard deviation and, for example, a reliability of 0.8, the error of measurement associated with any individual score is 45 per cent of the standard deviation. With a reliability of 0.5, the standard error is 70 per cent of a standard deviation, so we have improved the precision of measurement by only 30 per cent over the information we would have prior to doing any assessment of the individual at all.

Another way to interpret this is to imagine that we had a scale with a standard deviation of 10 and a reliability of 0.8. If someone's true score were 15 on the measure, then we would expect that 68 per cent of the time her observed score would fall between $15 - (10 \times 0.45)$ and $15 + (10 \times 0.45)$, i.e. between 10.5 and 19.5.

Expected difference in scores on retesting

If a person takes the same test on two occasions, how big a difference in test scores can be expected? The standard deviation of the difference between two scores is $\sqrt{2} \times$ SEM. Modifying the previous example slightly, imagine we have a test where the person's *observed* score was 15 and the SEM was 3. As we just saw, the probability is 68 per cent that the true score is between 12 and 18. If the person takes the test a second time, then the probability is 68 per cent that the second score will be somewhere within the interval of $15 - (\sqrt{2} \times 3)$ and $15 + (\sqrt{2} \times 3)$, or between 10.8 and 19.2. The interval is larger because there will be some error in both the first and the second observed scores, whereas in determining the interval in which the true score lies, there is error involved only for the observed score, but not for the true one (Green 1981).

Empirical data on retest reliability

One way of evaluating the adequacy of reliability coefficients obtained from a new instrument is to compare them against tests which are generally assumed to have acceptable levels. Schuerger *et al.* (1982) and Schuerger *et al.* (1989) compiled data from a number of personality questionnaires, readministered over intervals ranging from two days to 20 years. Scales which tap relatively stable traits, such as extraversion, have test–retest coefficients in the high 0.70s to low 0.80s when readministered within the same year, dropping to the mid-0.60s over a 20 year span. Measures of mild and presumably variable pathological states, such as anxiety, have coefficients about 0.10 lower than trait measures. Conversely, IQ tests, especially when administered to adults, have retest reliabilities about 0.10 higher (Schuerger and Witt 1989). Some measures of competence, specifically specialty certification examinations, have been shown to have similar correlations of about 0.70 over a seven to 10 year interval (Ramsey *et al.* 1989).

Standards for the magnitude of the reliability coefficient

From the previous sections, it should be evident that reliability cannot be conceived of as a property which a particular instrument does or does not possess;

rather, any measure will have a certain degree of reliability when applied to certain populations under certain conditions. The issue which must be addressed is how much reliability is 'good enough'. Authors of textbooks on psychometric theory often make brief recommendations, usually without justification or reference to other recommendations. In fact, there can be no sound basis for such a recommendation, any more than there can be a sound basis for the decision that a certain percentage of candidates sitting an examination will fail.

For what it is worth, here are two authors' opinions for acceptable reliability for tests used to make a decision about individuals: Kelley (1927) recommended a minimum of 0.94, while Weiner and Stewart (1984) suggested 0.85.

Fortunately, some authors avoid any such arbitrary judgement. However, the majority of textbooks then make a further distinction: namely, that a test used for individual judgement should be more reliable than one used for group decisions or research purposes. There are two possible justifications for this distinction. First, the research will draw conclusions from a mean score averaged across many individuals, and the sample size will serve to reduce the error of measurement in comparison to group differences. Second, rarely will decisions about research findings be made on the basis of a single study; conclusions are usually drawn from a series of replicated studies. But a recommendation of reliability, such as attempted by Weiner and Stewart (1984), remains tenuous since a sample of 1000 can tolerate a much less reliable instrument than a sample of 10, so that the acceptable reliability is dependent on the sample size used in the research.

Reliability and the probability of misclassification

An additional problem of interpretation arising from the reliability coefficient is that it does not, of itself, indicate just how many wrong decisions (false positives or false negatives) will result from a measure with a particular reliability. There is no straightforward answer to this problem, since the probability of misclassification, when the underlying measure is continuous, relates both to the property of the instrument and to the decision of the location of the cut point. For example, if we had people trained to assess haemoglobin using an office haemoglobinometer and classify patients as normal or anaemic on the basis of a single random blood sample, the number of false positives and false negatives will be dependent on the reliability of the reading of a single sample, but will also depend on two other variables: where we decide to set the boundary between normal and anaemic, and the base rate of anaemia in the population under study.

Clearly there must be some relationship between the reliability of the scores and the likelihood that the decision will result in a misclassification. Some indication of the relationship between reliability and the probability of misclassification was given by Thorndike and Hagen (1969), who avoided the 'cut point' problem by examining the ranking of individuals. Imagine 100 people who have been tested and ranked. Consider one individual ranked 25th from the top, and another ranked 50th. If the reliability is 0, there is a 50 per cent chance that the two will reverse order on repeated testing since the measure conveys no information and the ordering, as a result, is arbitrary. With a reliability of 0.5, there is still a 37 per cent chance of reversal; a reliability of 0.8 will result in 20 per cent reversals; and 0.95 will result in their reversing order 2.2 per cent of the time. From this example, it is evident that reliability of 0.75 is a fairly minimal requirement for a useful instrument.

Improving reliability

If we return to the basic definition of reliability as a ratio of subject variance to subject + error variance, we can improve reliability only by increasing the magnitude of the variance between subjects relative to the error variance. This can be accomplished in a number of ways, both legitimate and otherwise.

There are several approaches to reducing error variance. Many authors recommend observer training, although the specific strategies to be used in training raters are usually unspecified. Alternatively, Newble *et al.* (1980) have suggested that observers have difficulty acquiring new skills. They recommend, as a result, that if consistently extreme observers are discovered, they simply be eliminated from further use. The strategies for improving scale design discussed in Chapter 4 may also contribute to reducing error variance.

Similarly, there are a number of ways of enhancing the true variance. If the majority of individual scores are either very high or very low, so that the average score is approaching the maximum or minimum possible (the 'ceiling' or 'floor'), then many of the items are being wasted. The solution is to introduce items that will result in performance nearer the middle of the scale, effectively increasing true variance. One could also modify the descriptions on the scale; for example, by changing 'poor—fair—good—excellent' to 'fair—good—very good—excellent'.

An alternative approach, which is *not* legitimate, is to administer the test to a more heterogeneous group of subjects for the purpose of determining reliability. For example, if a measure of function in arthritis does not reliably discriminate among ambulatory arthritics, administering the test to both normal subjects and to bedridden hospitalized arthritics will almost certainly improve reliability. Of course, the resulting reliability no longer yields any information about the ability of the instrument to discriminate among ambulatory patients.

By contrast, it is sometimes the case that a reliability coefficient derived from a homogeneous population is to be applied to a population which is more heterogeneous. It is clear from the above discussion that the reliability in the application envisioned will be larger than that determined in the homogeneous study population. If the standard deviations of the two samples are known, it is poss-

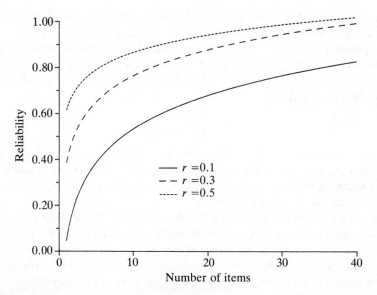

Fig. 8.3. Relation between number of items and reliability.

ible to calculate a new reliability coefficient, or to *correct for attenuation*, using the following formula:

$$R_{revised} = \frac{R \times \sigma^2_{new}}{R \times \sigma^2_{new} + (1 - R) \times \sigma^2_{old}}$$

where σ^2_{new} and σ^2_{old} are the variances of the new and original samples, respectively, and R is the original reliability.

Perhaps the simplest way to improve reliability is to increase the number of items on the test. It is not self-evident why this should help, but the answer lies in statistical theory. As long as the test items are not perfectly correlated, the true variance will increase as the square of the number of items, whereas the error variance will increase only as the number of items. So, if the test length is tripled, true variance will be nine times as large, and error variance three times as large as the original test, as long as the new items are similar psychometrically to the old ones. From the Spearman-Brown formula, which we discussed in Chapter 5, the new reliability will be:

$$R_{SB} = \frac{3 \times R}{1 + 2 \times R}$$

If the original reliability was 0.7, the tripled test will have a reliability of 0.875. The relationship between the number of items and test length is shown in Figure 8.3.

In practice, the equation tends to overestimate the new reliability, since we tend to think up (or 'borrow') the easier, more obvious items first. When we have to devise new items, they often are not as good as the original ones.

The Spearman-Brown formula can be used in another way. If we know the reliability of a test of a particular length is r and we wish to achieve a reliability of R, then the formula can be modified to indicate the factor by which we must increase the test length, k:

$$k = \frac{R(1-r)}{r(1-R)}$$

To improve measures of stability, such as test–retest reliability, one can always shorten the retest interval. However, if the instrument is intended to measure states of duration of weeks or months, the demonstration of retest reliability over hours or days is not useful.

Finally, it is evident from the foregoing discussion that there is not a single reliability associated with a measure. A more useful approach to the issue of reliability is to critically examine the components of variance due to each source of variation in turn, and then focus efforts on reducing the larger sources of error variance. This approach, called *generalizability theory*, is covered in the next chapter.

Sample size estimation for reliability studies

In conducting a reliability study, we are attempting to estimate the reliability coefficient with as much accuracy as possible; that is, we want to be certain that the true reliability coefficient is reasonably close to the estimate we have determined. This is one form of the *confidence interval* (for further discussion consult one of the recommended statistics books). As we might expect, the larger the sample size, the smaller will be the confidence interval. Confidence interval formulae for intraclass correlations are quite complex, and difficult to use for sample size estimation. However, we can approximate the bounds on the ICC by using formulae derived for the Pearson correlation. Even here, we cannot calculate the confidence interval (CI) around the correlation directly, since the distribution of r is not normal. It is first necessary to normalize it using Fisher's z' transformation, where:

$$z'(r) = \frac{1}{2} \log_e \frac{(1+r)}{(1-r)}$$

and half of the confidence interval (CI_H) is:

$$z'(r) + z_{\alpha/2} \frac{1}{N-3}$$

N is therefore:

$$N = \left[\frac{z_{\alpha/2}}{z'(r) - z'(r + CI_H)} \right]^2 + 3$$

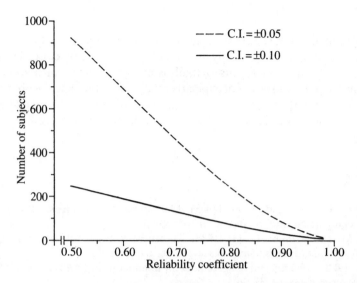

Fig. 8.4. Sample sizes for reliability studies.

where $z_{\alpha/2}$ = 1.96 for a 95 per cent CI and 2.54 for a 99 per cent CI. Thus, the width of the CI depends on the correlation: larger when r is small and smaller when r is close to 1. Figure 8.4 can be used to estimate N for an α of 0.05, and CI_{HS} of 0.05 and 0.10. Since sample size estimation is only an approximate 'science' (because the size of the reliability coefficient and the width of the CI are merely best guesses), the graph should be accurate enough for most purposes. If a more precise estimate is needed (or the coefficient is less than 0.50), you can use either the equation or the table in Streiner (1994).

This approach differs from that taken by other authors (e.g. Donner and Eliasziw 1987), who base the calculation on the number of subjects needed to determine if the coefficient is significantly different from some arbitrary value. In most instances, this is not the question we are asking; we are usually more interested in estimating the magnitude of the reliability coefficient, rather than seeing if it is statistically significantly different from some other value.

Still another approach to estimating the sample size is to use a fixed number. Thus, Nunnally (1978) recommends that the study involve at least 300 subjects, while Guilford (1956) and Kline (1986) are a little less demanding and recommend 200 subjects. However, these suggestions do not take into account the fact that for a confidence interval of a given width, the sample size varies with the magnitude of the coefficient. So, for a CI_H of 0.10 (with α = 0.05), Nunnally's recommendation would result in 'statistical overkill' for any coefficient greater than 0.18; and Guilford's and Kline's for any greater than 0.58. If we expected that the reliability coefficient would be 0.70, for example, the equation would yield a sample size requirement of only 130 subjects.

Summary

The discussion regarding appropriate measures of reliability is easily resolved. The Pearson correlation is theoretically incorrect but usually fairly close. The method of Altman and Bland is analogous (actually isomorphic) to the calculation of error variance in the ICC, and does not explicitly relate this to the range of observations. Thus we are left with kappa and the intraclass correlation, which yield identical results, so the choice can be dictated by ease of calculation, nothing else.

References

Altman, D. G. and Bland, J. M. (1983). Measurement in medicine: The analysis of method comparison studies. *Statistician*, **32**, 307–17.

Bland, J. M. and Altman, D. G. (1986). Statistical methods for assessing agreement between two methods of clinical measurement. *Lancet*, **i**, 307–10.

Cohen, J. (1960). A coefficient of agreement for nominal scales. *Educational and Psychological Measurement*, **20**, 37–46.

Cohen, J. (1968). Weighted kappa: Nominal scale agreement with provision for scaled disagreement or partial credit. *Psychological Bulletin*, **70**, 213–20.

Cronbach, L. J. (1957). The two disciplines of scientific psychology. *American Psychologist*, **12**, 671–84.

Donner, A. and Eliasziw, M. (1987). Sample size requirements for reliability studies. *Statistics in Medicine*, **6**, 441–8.

Fleiss, J. L. and Cohen, J. (1973). The equivalence of weighted kappa and the intraclass correlation coefficient as measures of reliability. *Educational and Psychological Measurement*, **33**, 613–19.

Green, B. F. (1981). A primer of testing. *American Psychologist*, **36**, 1001–11.

Guilford, J. P. (1956). *Psychometric methods* (2nd edn). McGraw Hill, New York.

Kelley, T. L. (1927). *Interpretation of educational measurements*. World Books, Yonkers.

Kline, P. (1986). *A handbook of test construction*. Methuen, London.

Newble, D. I., Hoare, J., and Sheldrake, P. F. (1980). The selection and training of examiners for clinical examinations. *Medical Education*, **4**, 345–9.

Norman, G. R. and Streiner, D. L. (1994). *Biostatistics: The bare essentials*. Mosby, St Louis, MO.

Nunnally, J. C. (1978). *Psychometric theory*. McGraw-Hill, New York.

Ramsey, P. G., Carline, J. D., Inui, T. S., Larson, E. B., LoGerfo, J. P., and Weinrich, M. D. (1989). Predictive validity of certification by the American Board of Internal Medicine. *Annals of Internal Medicine*, **110**, 719–26.

Schuerger, J. M. Tait, E., and Tavernelli, M. (1982). Temporal stability of personality by questionnaire. *Journal of Personality and Social Psychology*, **43**, 176–82.

Schuerger, J. M., and Witt, A. C. (1989). The temporal stability of individually tested intelligence. *Journal of Clinical Psychology*, **45**, 294–302.

Schuerger, J. M., Zarella, K. L., and Hotz, A. S. (1989). Factors that influence the temporal stability of personality by questionnaire. *Journal of Personality and Social Psychology*, **56**, 777–83.

Shrout, P. E. and Fleiss, J. L. (1979). Intraclass correlations: Uses in assessing rater reliability. *Psychological Bulletin*, **86**, 420–8.

Streiner, D. L. (1994). Sample size formulae for parameter estimation. *Perceptual and Motor Skills*, **78**, 275–84.

Thorndike, R. L. and Hagen, E. (1969). *Measurement and evaluation in education and psychology*. Wiley, New York.

Weiner, E. A. and Stewart, B. J. (1984). *Assessing individuals*. Little Brown, Boston.

9

Generalizability theory

Classical test theory, upon which the reliability coefficient is based, begins with a simple assumption—that an observed test score can be decomposed into two parts: a 'true' score (which no one really knows) and an 'error' score (i.e. $Score_{Observed} = Score_{True} + e$). As we discussed in the previous chapter, this assumption then leads directly to the formulation of the reliability coefficient as the ratio of true variance to (true + error) variance.

We saw that there are many approaches to estimating reliability, each of which generates a different coefficient. One can examine scores from the same observer on two viewings of the same stimulus (intra-observer), different observers of the same stimulus (inter-observer), different occasions separated by a short time interval (test–retest), different items (internal consistency), different forms of the scale (parallel forms), and so on. Further, these standard measures do not exhaust the possible sources of variance. For example, some measures such as bone density or tenderness might be expected to be equal on both sides of the body (left–right reliability?), and skin colour might be expected to be the same on the soles of hands and feet (top–bottom reliability?).

Clearly, the assumption that all variance in scores can be neatly divided into true and error variance is simplistic. Instead, for each person we have measured there are, in addition to the 'true' score of that individual, multiple potential sources of error. Our goal is to obtain the most precise estimate we can of the score that person should have if there were no sources of error contaminating our results; each of the multiple forms of reliability that we have mentioned identifies and quantifies only one source of error variance.

This may not, of itself, be problematic. Conceptually at least, we could consider a long series of studies, each of which determined one source of error variance. We could, perhaps, then put all of these error variances together to arrive at the appropriate reliability coefficients.

Unfortunately, in addition to the semi-infinite research agenda this would generate (those eager for tenure and promotion may view this as an advantage rather than a handicap), there are other flies in the ointment. Remember that we estimate the true score optimistically as the average across all the allowed observations. This strategy will inevitably lead to different estimates of true scores from each study, with no logical way to combine them. As one example, imagine we did an inter- and intra-rater reliability study with two observers and a seven point scale. Assume that one observer used the whole scale, but the other used only the points from 3 to 5, and that their individual judgements were almost perfectly reproducible. Both intra-rater studies would result in the same near-zero error variance; however, the subject variance of one study would be about four times as large as the other, leading to very different estimates of 'the' reliability.

Finally, there may be interactions amongst the sources of error variance. We will use the Objective Structured Clinical Examination (OSCE; Harden and Gleeson 1979) as an example. In it, students rotate through a series of 'stations', typically of 5–10 minutes duration each, where they perform a component of a clinical examination such as taking a brief history of abdominal pain from a simulated patient, physically examining a chest, or interpreting a radiograph. Although some stations, such as the radiographic interpretation, may be unobserved and scored later, clinical stations are more typically observed and scored by clinician examiners. If we did an inter-observer reliability study on each station using two independent examiners, we would create a whole set of reliability coefficients, one for each station. We could also do an 'inter-station reliability study', examining the correlation across stations. But to the extent that examiners are chosen with expertise in particular skills, and have different scoring styles, the amount of error variance may differ from station to station, amounting to a subject by examiner by station component of variance, which cannot be captured from the individual studies. What we really need is some way of combining all the sources of variability in a single study, using all the data to estimate the variance between subjects and the various components of error variance.

This broad approach was originally devised by Cronbach and his associates and is known as *generalizability theory* (Cronbach *et al.* 1972). The essence of the theory is the recognition that in any measurement situation there are multiple (in fact, infinite) sources of error variance. An important goal of measurement is to attempt to identify, measure, and thereby find strategies to reduce the influence of these sources on the measurement in question. Although the theory is now over 20 years old, it is only within the last few years that it has become a routine approach to measurement in the health sciences. A few review articles have appeared which elaborate on, or utilize, the concepts of generalizability theory (Boodoo and O'Sullivan 1982; Evans *et al.* 1981; Shavelson *et al.* 1989; van der Vleuten and Swanson 1990).

Imagine that we could identify the most likely sources of error in a measurement of some characteristic of a person. Having made this step (e.g. declaring that the important sources of error in this measurement situation were the observer, the time of day, and the phase of the moon), we have then defined our 'universe' of possible observations to include different observers, morning, noon and night, and four lunar phases. If we then proceeded to average each person's scores over all these possible conditions, this would be an unbiased estimate of that person's score over the universe as we have defined it. Note that there is no pretence that this is a 'true' score, since we may well have guessed wrong about the universe—maybe it's the phases of Mars, not the moon, that really matter—but this is still a best guess at a 'universe' score for our predefined and finite universe of observations.

G Studies

Presuming that we have done a reasonable job of identifying the possible sources of error, these would then be incorporated into a research design, called a *generalizability study* or '*G study*', where all the sources are contained as repeated measures on each subject. The next step then would be to use the data we have gathered to determine the extent to which each of these variables actually influenced the score. One way of expressing this variability is to use the concepts of analysis of variance, as we did in Chapter 8. Thus, to the extent that the time of day does influence the obtained scores, then the analysis of the data will show that the variance due to time will be large relative to other components. As we pointed out already, if the sources we have identified are trivial, and we have missed some important sources of error, then there will be a large amount of variance due to *random error* or *residual*. By identifying these sources of error, we can determine the relative importance of each component in adding error to a measurement. In turn, this information can then lead to specific strategies to reduce major components of error and improve measurement, the details of which will be discussed later.

Once we have determined all the sources of variance, we can then construct appropriate coefficients reflecting different decision situations. For example, we can create a coefficient showing the extent to which we can generalize from observations made by one observer on one day in one lunar phase to another observation made by another observer on the same day in the same phase, the equivalent of the standard inter-rater reliability. In the terminology of generalizability theory, 'observer' is a *facet of generalization*, and since we wish to differentiate among patients, 'patient' is a *facet of differentiation*. Lunar phase and day, since they are fixed, are called *fixed facets*. Another coefficient may be determined by keeping the observer fixed but generalizing across days; here the facet of differentiation is still patients, the facet of generalization is days, and the fixed facets are observer and lunar phase. This is, of course, the equivalent of 'intra-rater' or 'test–retest' reliability.

D studies

Having generated the variance estimates, we can then determine the effect of changing the number of observations. For instance, we can see what will happen to the generalizability coefficient if we add a third observer, or decrease the number of days of observation from four to three. Since these explore the impact

Table 9.1 *Assessment of ten patients by three physiotherapists on two days*

Patient	Observer 1		Observer 2		Observer 3	
	Day 1	Day 5	Day 1	Day 5	Day 1	Day 5
1						
2						
.						
.						
.						
10						

of certain decisions, they are called *Decision* or *D studies*. These 'studies' are done using only paper and pencil (or a computer), dividing each term by the new number of observations in each facet. This then permits us to see what we must do to increase the reliability to an acceptable level, or conversely, how much the reliability will decline if we make the real-life situation more feasible by eliminating testings.

Within generalizability theory, the patient or subject no longer has any special status. For example, we may want to know the extent to which the scores can differentiate among sadness states related to different phases of the moon. For this D study, lunar phase is the facet of differentiation, patient is the facet of generalization, and observer and day are fixed facets. (This example is not as bizarre as it may first appear. Much effort has been expended trying to relate psychiatric admissions to the full moon, and even to sun-spot activity.)

It is evident that the conventional approaches to reliability—test–retest, inter-observer, and so on—become simply special cases of a more general formulation which seeks to identify the important sources of variance in a particular measurement situation from the outset, and then attempts to quantify these sources of error.

Example 1—Therapists, Occasions, and Patients

An example may clarify the theory. Imagine a group of respiratory patients enrolled in a rehabilitation program. In order to determine the reliability of measurement of pulmonary function, three physiotherapists make independent assessments on two successive visits five days apart. The design may look like Table 9.1.

It is evident that this design contains elements of both inter-observer and test–retest reliability. To the extent that the scores assigned by various therapists on the same day differ, this will contribute to a reduction in inter-observer reliabi-

Table 9.2 *Analysis of variance table*

Source	Sum of squares	d.f.	Mean square (MS)	Expected mean square (EMS)
Patients (p)	3915	9	435	$\sigma^2_{dop} + 2\sigma^2_{op} + 3\sigma^2_{dp} + 6\sigma^2_p$
Day (d)	815	1	815	$\sigma^2_{dop} + 3\sigma^2_{dp} + 10\sigma^2_{do} + 30\sigma^2_d$
Day × Patients (dp)	585	9	65	$\sigma^2_{dop} + 3\sigma^2_{dp}$
Observer (o)	960	2	480	$\sigma^2_{dop} + 2\sigma^2_{op} + 10\sigma^2_{do} + 20\sigma^2_o$
Observer × Patients (op)	540	18	30	$\sigma^2_{dop} + 2\sigma^2_{op}$
Day × Observer (do)	340	2	170	$\sigma^2_{dop} + 10\sigma^2_{do}$
Day × Observer × Patients (dop)	360	18	20	σ^2_{dop}

lity. Observations by the *same* observer on the second occasion are a measure of test–retest reliability.

What makes this design approach different from conventional assessment is that both sources of error (therapist and occasion) are incorporated in the *same* design, instead of conducting two separate studies. This tactic has three methodological advantages. First, subject or patient variance is a single estimate using all the data. Second, the estimate of each reliability is derived from multiple observations, since three raters are contributing to the assessment of test–retest reliability, and two occasions are summed together to yield a measure of inter-observer reliability. This effectively increases the sample size and thereby improves precision. Third, combining the two sources of variation into one experiment permits the consideration of additional combinations of error variance. For example, it is likely that our real concern is the reliability of an observation made by *any* therapist on *any* occasion, a situation which would suggest the need for a test–retest/inter-observer reliability coefficient. This coefficient can be easily determined from a design such as that in the example, but would not normally be available from applications of classical test theory.

Continuing with the example, we might explore how the various components of variance are derived. For simplicity, we limit ourselves to the two-factor case, including only variation due to multiple observers and repeated occasions of observation. If the data were analysed using repeated-measures ANOVA, the results would resemble Table 9.2.

Note that this table includes the expected mean squares, expressed as a sum of variance components. The detailed derivation of these expressions can be found

Table 9.3 *Components of variance*

Source	Variance
Patients	60
Day	20
Day × Patients	15
Observer	15
Observer × Patients	5
Day × Observer	15
Day × Observer × Patients	20

in statistics texts (e.g. Glass and Stanley 1970), so we will just give a brief indication of the conceptual basis of the expressions.

The basic notation of the mean square (MS) as a sum of variances was discussed in Chapter 8. Every MS contains both the variance due to the factor of interest and also variance due to all other sources which interact with it; so for example, the MS due to observers contains variance due to observers, and also variance due to the interaction between observers and patients, observers and days, and observers, days, and patients (which is just the residual error term in this example). At first sight, this seems nonsensical, since we have already separately calculated the variance due to all the other interactions. However, the apparent contradiction resides in the basic assumption of statistics which distinguishes between samples and populations. The MS terms we have calculated are *estimates* of the population variances, expressed in σ^2 terms. Even if, for example, there really was no difference between observers, or no 'main effect' of observers, we might expect that random fluctuations would result in some difference between the calculated means for each observer, and hence some non-zero value of the MS due to observers. The extent to which this calculated MS differs from the population variance due to observers is imbedded in the magnitude of the interaction terms, and thus these interactions contribute to the expected MS.

Furthermore, each MS is actually summed up over all levels of the factors *not* contained in the expression; the *DP* interaction is summed over the three levels of the observer, and the *O* main effect is summed over the 10 levels of patients and two levels of days. As a result, when these variance components are entered into the expected mean square (EMS) expression, they contain multipliers accounting for the levels of the factors *not* in each term.

Further elaboration of the derivation of these expressions is beyond the scope of this book. Suffice it to say that from these formulae we can derive the resulting variance components. These are shown above in Table 9.3.

From this analysis, it is apparent that the main source of variance in the measurements is *P*, which indicates that most of the variability in the measurements is due to systematic differences between patients. This is the expectation, and indicates that we were successful in discriminating among patients. Relatively less variance is due to the main effects of D (suggesting systematically higher or lower values on different days) and O (reflecting systematic differences between observers). The DP interaction shows that some patients did better on day 1 than day 5, while this was reversed for other patients. The OD interaction is interpreted in a similar manner. The low variance due to the OP interaction is encouraging, reflecting that the observers' ratings are *not* influenced by specific patients. Finally, the residual (DOP) interaction is relatively large (20) in comparison to the remaining sources of variance, possibly suggesting that there are other important factors we might have included in the G study.

Applying the approaches of the previous chapter, we could easily conjure up a reliability coefficient consisting of the variance due to patients (60), divided by the sum of all the variance components (150), or 0.4. Unfortunately, this approach simply indicates that the other factors are contributing considerable error variance, but does not indicate where it came from or how one might improve the situation.

Let us examine Table 9.3 in more detail. First, note that the main effects of D and O imply simply that the average score on day 1 differed from the score on day 5, and that there were differences in the average scores of the observers. This may be of no consequence if we simply wish to compare scores on the same day or by the same observer, or alternatively if we are willing to apply a correction factor to eliminate this source of bias in each estimate. Conversely, the interaction terms between P and the other variables represent the extent to which each source directly contributes *random* variation to a score. For example, the OP interaction implies that some patients are rated differently by some observers than by other observers, an effect that we cannot disentangle if we wish to use scores obtained from different observers. However, this interaction term is irrelevant if we wish to look only at the reliability of the ratings by the same observer on successive days. In this case, the DP interaction term expresses the amount of random error in repeated scores by the same observer.

These observations suggest that it may be possible to use the variance components identified in the analysis of variance to construct a series of coefficients which will depend on the variables which will remain constant (or 'fixed') in a particular measurement situation, and the variables one wishes to make generalizations over.

Continuing with this example, suppose we want to use these data to examine inter-observer reliability. In this case, the fact that the observations were repeated on two occasions is incidental; what we want to focus on is differences between observers. The design looks as if we had done an inter-observer reliability study twice.

In examining inter-observer reliability, then, the change in scores that occurred with the passage of time is incidental, and so the main effect of day would be excluded from the sources of variance in this generalizability coefficient. Second, if the day factor were not explicitly calculated as a variance component, then the interaction between day and patients would end up in the sum of squares due to patients. So if we wish to calculate the coefficient equivalent to an inter-observer reliability, the numerator would contain the main effect of patients, and the interaction between patients and day.

Extrapolating from this example, then, in constructing a generalizability coefficient, the numerator of the coefficient contains the variance due to patients and all interactions between patients and any factors over which one does not wish to generalize (such as day). The denominator contains variance due to patients, interactions between patients and all other factors, and the random error term (in this case, patient × observer × day). The generalizability coefficient becomes:

$$\frac{\sigma^2_P + \sigma^2_{DP}}{\sigma^2_P + \sigma^2_{OP} + \sigma^2_{DP} + \sigma^2_{DOP}} = \frac{60 + 15}{60 + 5 + 15 + 20} = 0.75.$$

In looking at the test–retest reliability, the opposite situation arises. In this circumstance, variance due to systematic differences between observers (i.e. the main effect of O) is irrelevant. Analogously, the OP interaction is incorporated into the variance due to patients in the numerator of the coefficient. So, the generalizability coefficient becomes:

$$\frac{\sigma^2_P + \sigma^2_{OP}}{\sigma^2_P + \sigma^2_{OP} + \sigma^2_{DP} + \sigma^2_{DOP}} = \frac{60 + 5}{60 + 5 + 15 + 20} = 0.65.$$

Finally, one may wish to generalize from a rating by one observer on one day to a rating by a different observer at another time. This coefficient has no classical equivalent, and equals:

$$\frac{\sigma^2_P}{\sigma^2_P + \sigma^2_{OP} + \sigma^2_{DP} + \sigma^2_{DOP}} = \frac{60}{60 + 5 + 15 + 20} = 0.60.$$

As one would expect, this coefficient is lower than either of the preceding ones.

This example provides some insight into the nature of generalizability theory. The approach begins by attempting to define all the significant sources of observational error—observers, days, items, and so forth. These are then incorporated into a factorial experimental design, and components of variance determined. Different coefficients can then be calculated depending on which factors ('facets' in the theory) will remain fixed and which will vary.

The example we used was based on a simple ANOVA design, in which there were two factors, and each factor occurred at all levels of the other factors: a 'crossed' design in the language of analysis of variance. However, the method can be used with more complex designs, including as many as four or five factors, as well as 'nested' designs, where the factor structure is more complex. The general approach remains the same; to begin by isolating the various sources of variance in the scores, and then generating a family of coefficients which depend on the particular factors which are allowed to vary and remain fixed.

D study examples

Having obtained the estimates of variance coefficients, we are now in the position to estimate a wide range of D coefficients to address various possible decision situations. While some of these may be performed by the investigator as part of the original study, the fact that there are estimates of variance components available enables the reader to construct additional G coefficients corresponding to his or her decision situation.

For example, given the clinical situation we began with where patients are being assessed on multiple occasions over the course of treatment, it might be reasonable to determine whether we get a more reliable estimate of different patients' disease by using multiple therapists rating the patient on a single day, or one therapist rating the patient over several days. We noted in our previous example that the observer was a relatively small source of variance compared to the day of assessment. Therefore, the logically more appropriate strategy would appear to be to take assessments on several days using a single observer. The alternative strategy of gathering observations from multiple observers on a single day would provide relatively little gain.

The effect of these strategies can be quantified. Since the variance of the average of n observations is just the initial variance divided by n, this can be included in the generalizability coefficients. Let us compare the following two strategies:

(a) one observer on three successive days

     vs.

(b) three observers on a single day.

For case (a), the variance due to days × patients and the error variance will be reduced by a factor of 3, so the new coefficient is:

$$G = \frac{60}{60 + 5 + \frac{15}{3} + \frac{15}{3}} = 0.78.$$

Similarly, the coefficient for the second strategy will have the observer × patients interaction and the error variance divided by 3, to result in:

$$G = \frac{60}{60 + \frac{5}{3} + 15 + \frac{20}{3}} = 0.72.$$

Therefore the second strategy resulted in a lower coefficient, even though it used the same amount of therapist time.

We have also stated that there can be different facets of differentiation, and patient is only one possibility. In the present example we might, for instance, ascertain whether the instrument can distinguish among therapists, determining those who are systematically lower or higher in their estimates; information which might be useful in deciding whether to initiate a training programme for therapists. More interesting, perhaps, is the use of generalizability theory to distinguish between the two occasions of assessment, on the first and fifth day. We might have expected some response to therapy after five days of treatment; the question is whether the measure can detect this effect.

There is a large literature devoted to the measurement of change, and Chapter 11 discusses many of these issues in detail. In the present situation, we simply wish to demonstrate that the measurement of change is a natural aspect of generalizability theory, and the creation of a 'responsiveness to change coefficient' is just one more variation on the central theme. In this case, the facet of differentiation is day (to what extent can we differentiate among different days of treatment?), the facet of generalization is patient (to what extent does the change from day 1 to day 5 generalize across patients?) and observer is the fixed facet.

The appropriate G coefficient now is:

$$G = \frac{\sigma^2_D + \sigma^2_{DO}}{\sigma^2_D + \sigma^2_{DO} + \sigma^2_{DP} + \sigma^2_{DOP}} = \frac{20 + 15}{20 + 15 + 15 + 20} = 0.50$$

Thus, the G coefficient related to responsiveness is very similar to the reliability coefficient; in fact, two of the terms in the denominator are identical.

Example 2—Items, Observers, and Stations – the OSCE

In this example, we will use the OSCE format, which we discussed earlier, to illustrate the idea of 'nested' factors. We presume that each examiner will be rating students at only one station, and second, that the rating form used at each station is specific to the station, although the number of categories is the same for all stations (to ease computation and interpretation). For example, each examiner may complete a global rating on a seven point scale for each of three different dimensions (e.g. completeness of history taking, and accuracy of the physical examination). Let us suppose that there are two observers per case, four stations, and 10 students. Thus, in G theory terminology, the universe of observations consists of four facets: the observer, with two levels, the rating, with three levels; the station or case, with four levels; and the student, with 10 levels. To complicate things further, since each observer stays at one station for the exercise, observer is 'nested' within case. Second, since each station examines a different aspect of competence, the four ratings in each station may in turn address different aspects on each station, so rating is also nested within case. The study design is shown in Table 9.4.

Because the observer and the rating are nested within each case, we cannot examine the interaction between these factors and the case. This results in fewer lines in the ANOVA table, and some more complications in the estimated mean squares. For a sample of data we used, the ANOVA table looked like Table 9.5.

Now the next step, as usual, is to derive formulae for the expected mean squares. Again, the approach is complicated but is presented in some statistics

Table 9.4   *Design of a typical OSCE with four stations, two observers and three ratings*

Student	Station 1		Station 2		...	Station 4	
	Obs 1	Obs 2	Obs 3	Obs4	...	Obs 7	Obs 8
1	R_1 R_2 R_3	R_1 R_2 R_3	R_1 R_2 R_3	R_1 R_2 R_3	...	R_1 R_2 R_3	R_1 R_2 R_3
2					...		
3					...		
4					...		
5					...		
.							
.							
10					...		

Table 9.5   *ANOVA table for example 2*

Source	Sum of squares	df	Mean square
Student S	85.23	9	9.47
Observer O:			
(C)	14.56	4	3.64
Rating R:(C)	11.00	4	1.37
Case C	118.48	3	39.49
S × O(C)	111.76	36	3.10
S × R(C)	70.33	72	0.98
S × C	205.93	27	7.62
O × C	6.93	8	0.87
S × O × R(C)	61.73	72	0.86
Error			

Table 9.6 *Estimated mean squares and variances for example 2*

Source	Expected mean square	Calculated Variance
Student S	$\sigma^2_{Err} + 6\sigma^2_{SC} + 3\sigma^2_{SO(C)} + 2\sigma^2_{SR(C)} + 24\sigma^2_S$	0.077
Observer O: (C)	$\sigma^2_{Err} + 3\sigma^2_{SO(C)} + 10\sigma^2_{SR(C)} + 30\sigma^2_{O(C)}$	0.017
Rating R: (C)	$\sigma^2_{Err} + 2\sigma^2_{SO(C)} + 10\sigma^2_{OR(C)} + 20\sigma^2_{r(C)}$	0.019
Case C	$\sigma^2_{Err} + 2\sigma^2_{SR(C)} + 10\sigma^2_{OR(C)} + 3\sigma^2_{SO(C)}$ $+ 6\sigma^2_{SC} + 20\sigma^2_{R(C)} + 30\sigma^2_{O(C)} + 60\sigma^2_C$	0.516
S × O(C)	$\sigma^2_{Err} + 3\sigma^3_{SO(C)}$	0.749
S × R(C)	$\sigma^2_{Err} + 2\sigma^2_{SR(C)}$	0.059
S × C	$\sigma^2_{Err} + 2\sigma^2_{SR(C)} + 3\sigma^2_{SO(C)} + 6\sigma^2_{SC}$	0.734
O × R	$\sigma^2_{Err} + 10\sigma^2_{OR(C)}$	0.001
S × O × R(C)	σ^2_{Err}	0.857

books. These, and the variances calculated from the mean squares using these formulas, are presented in Table 9.6.

Once the variances are computed, we can construct the appropriate G coefficients using the usual strategy. Thus, for differentiating among students, the denominator is always the same:

$$\text{Denominator 1} = \sigma^2_{SR(C)} + \sigma^2_{SC} + \sigma^2_{SO(C)} + \sigma^2_S + \sigma^2_{SOR(C)} = 2.476.$$

For generalization across ratings (a measure of the average inter-item correlation), case and observer are fixed factors, hence end up in the numerator with the main effect of students, so the coefficient is:

$$G(Ratings) = \frac{\sigma^2_{SC} + \sigma^2_{SO(C)} + \sigma^2_S}{\text{Denominator 1}} = \frac{1.560}{2.476} = 0.63.$$

This in turn may be modified into the equivalent of a Cronbach's alpha by dividing the appropriate error and interaction terms (those involving rating) by the number of ratings, three. So the new denominator is:

$$\text{Denominator 2} = \sigma^2_{SC} + \sigma^2_{SO(C)} + \sigma^2_{SR(C)}/3 + \sigma^2_S + \sigma^2_{SOR(C)}/3 =$$

$$1.866$$

and the G coefficient is now:

$$G(Ratings) = \frac{\sigma^2_{SC} + \sigma^2_{SO(C)} + \sigma^2_S}{\text{Denominator 2}} = \frac{1.560}{1.866} = 0.836$$

Similarly, the G coefficient for generalizing across observer, i.e. the inter-rater reliability, keeps rating and case as fixed factors, so the coefficient is:

$$G(Observer) = \frac{\sigma^2_{SC} + \sigma^2_{SR(C)} + \sigma^2_S}{\text{Denominator 1}} = \frac{0.870}{2.476} = 0.351.$$

For generalization across cases, we use the same strategy, keeping observer and rating as fixed factors:

$$G(Cases) = \frac{\sigma^2_{SO(C)} + \sigma^2_{SR(C)} + \sigma^2_{s}}{Denominator\ 1} = \frac{0.885}{2.476} = 0.357.$$

Finally, since OSCEs are frequently used in examination settings, the overall reliability of the test, which amounts to treating observer, rating, and case all as facets of generalization but dividing by the appropriate ns in order to determine the generalizability of the total test score, becomes:

$$G(Test) = \frac{\sigma^2_{s}}{\dfrac{\sigma^2_{SOR(C)}}{6} + \dfrac{\sigma^2_{SC}}{4} + \dfrac{\sigma^2_{SO(C)}}{2} + \dfrac{\sigma^2_{SR(C)}}{3} + \sigma^2_{s}} = \frac{0.077}{0.797} = 0.097$$

As we can see, from a design such as this, we can estimate all the conventional coefficients, using all the data in turn. The inclusion of appropriate nested factors complicates the ANOVA and the estimation of expected mean squares, but the calculation of variances and G coefficients, while messy, is completely analogous to the previous examples.

Example 3—Econometric *vs.* Psychometric Perspectives on the Utility of Health States

We described the standard econometric approaches to measurement in Chapter 4. A series of descriptions of health states are created, then a group of people— patients or non-patients—are approached and asked to rate the utility of the state, using standard gambles, time trade-offs, or other methods. The goal of measurement in these circumstances is to obtain a precise estimate of the utility of the various health states, so that resources can be appropriately allocated; in short, to differentiate among health states.

At least, that is the economist's goal. However, the same approach could conceivably be used to find out information about the raters; for example, whether the technique can identify consistent differences among raters which may be related to other characteristics such as depression, optimism, illness behaviour, etc. In this case, we are using the method to differentiate among raters. Finally, it has been of continuing interest to determine whether patients and non-patients rate the health states similarly (e.g. Sackett and Torrance 1978).

All of these questions fit naturally into a G theory framework. The design one might use involves three facets: health state (H), patient/non-patient (P), and rater nested within patient (R). Using, for example, 10 health states, and three raters nested within each status (since someone cannot be a patient and a non-patient, at least at the same time), the design may look like Table 9.7.

We have analysed the design using some artificial data, resulting in the ANOVA table in Table 9.8. The expected mean squares are not too complex,

Table 9.7 *Design for an econometric and psychometric G study*

State	Patient			Non-patient		
	R_1	R_2	R_3	R_4	R_5	R_6
1						
2						
3						
4						
.	.	.	.	.	.	.
.		.	.	.	.	.
9						
10						

Table 9.8 *ANOVA table for Example 3*

Source	Sum of squares	df	Mean square	Expected mean square	Variance
Health H	89.08	9	9.89	$\sigma^2_{Err} + 3\sigma^2_{HP} + 6\sigma^2_{H}$	1.39
Patient P non-patient	10.41	1	10.41	$\sigma^2_{Err} + 3\sigma^2_{HP} + 10\sigma^2_{R(P)} + 3\sigma^2_{P}$	0.31
Rater R(P)	1.73	4	0.43	$\sigma^2_{Err} + 10\sigma^2_{R(P)}$	0.00
H × P	13.75	9	1.52	$\sigma^2_{Err} + 3\sigma^2_{HP}$	0.21
H × R(P)	32.26	36	0.89	σ^2_{Err}	0.89

and we have solved these equations for the variance components in the same table. From our above discussion, the next step is to construct three different coefficients related to the three different perspectives. In this case, all the denominators may differ slightly as well as the numerators.

Perspective 1: Econometric

- Question: to what extent can we differentiate among health states, using ratings from patients and non-patients?
- Facet of differentiation: health

- Facet of generalization: patient, rater
- Coefficient:

$$G = \frac{\sigma^2_H}{\sigma^2_{H \times P} + \sigma^2_H + \sigma^2_{Err}} = \frac{1.39}{0.21 + 1.39 + 0.89} = 0.558.$$

Perspective 2: Psychometric

- Question: to what extent can we differentiate among individuals, regardless of patient status, using ratings of different health states?
- Facet of differentiation: rater
- Facet of generalization: patient, health
- Coefficient:

$$G = \frac{\sigma^2_{R(P)}}{\sigma^2_{R(P)} + \sigma^2_{Err}} = \frac{0.00}{0.00 + 0.89} = 0.000.$$

Perspective 3: Experimental

- Question: to what extent can we differentiate between non-patients and patients using ratings of health states?
- Facet of differentiation: patient/non-patient
- Facet of generalization: health, rater
- Coefficient:

$$G = \frac{\sigma^2_P}{\sigma^2_{H \times P} + \sigma^2_{R(P)} + \sigma^2_P + \sigma^2_{Err}} = \frac{0.31}{0.21 + 0.00 + 0.31 + 0.89} = 0.220.$$

It is clear that the success of this instrument is directly related to its intended use. It is reasonably good at differentiating among health states (particularly since we might use the G coefficient corresponding to the mean of all six ratings, which works out to 0.88); it is of very limited utility in differentiating between patients and non-patients; and it is completely useless in discriminating amongst individual raters.

Summary

Although generalizability theory is at first difficult to comprehend, the value of the method lies in the reinterpretation of the nature of measurement afforded by the theory. Instead of conceptualizing a measurement as a sum of a 'true' score and an 'error' score, generalizability theory forces a critical examination of the *sources* of measurement error. In addition, the effect of particular strategies to reduce error, based on multiple observations, can be directly estimated. As a result, the theory represents a powerful tool in advancing the methods of measurement.

References

Boodoo, G. M. and O'Sullivan, P. (1982). Obtaining generalizability coefficients for clinical evaluations. *Evaluation and the Health Professions*, **5**, 345–58.

Chambers, L. W., Haight, M., Norman, G. R., and MacDonald, L. (1987). Effect of mode of administration on a health status measure's responsiveness to change. *Medical Care*, **25**, 470–80.

Cronbach, L. J., Gleser, G. C., Nanda, H., and Rajaratnam, N. (1972). *The dependability of behavioral measurements: Theory of generalizability for scores and profiles.* Wiley, New York.

Evans, W. J., Cayten, C. G., and Green, P. A. (1981). Determining the generalizability of rating scales in clinical settings. *Medical Care*, **19**, 1211–19.

Glass, G. V. and Stanley, J. C. (1970). *Statistical methods in education and psychology.* Prentice-Hall, Englewood Cliffs, NJ.

Harden, R. M. and Gleeson, F. A. (1979). Assessment of clinical experience using an objective structured clinical examination (OSCE). *Medical Education*, **13**, 41–54.

Sackett, D. L. and Torrance, G. W. (1978). The utility of different health states as perceived by the general public. *Journal of Chronic Diseases*, **31**, 697–704.

Shavelson, R. J., Webb, N. M., and Rowley, G. L. (1989). Generalizability theory. *American Psychologist*, **44**, 922–32.

van der Vleuten, C. P. M. and Swanson D. B. (1990). Assessment of clinical skills with standardized patients: The state of the art. *Teaching and Learning in Medicine*, **2**, 58–76.

10

Validity

In the previous chapters, we examined various aspects of reliability; that is, how reproducible the results of a scale are under different conditions. This is a necessary step in establishing the usefulness of a measure, but it is not sufficient. The next step is to determine if the scale is measuring what we think it is; that is, the scale's *validity*. To illustrate the difference, imagine that we are trying to develop a new index to measure the degree of headache pain. We find that patients get the same score when they are tested on two different occasions, that different interviewers get similar results when assessing the same patient, and so on; in other words, the index is reliable. However, we still have no proof that differences in the total score reflect the degree of headache pain: the scale may be measuring pain from other sources; or it may be tapping factors entirely unrelated to pain, such as depression or the tendency to complain of bodily ailments. In this chapter, we will examine how to determine if we can draw valid conclusions from the scale.

Why assess validity?

The question that immediately arises is why we have to establish validity in the first place. After all, the health care fields are replete with measures that have never been 'validated' through any laborious testing process. Despite this, no one questions the usefulness of taking a patient's temperature to detect the presence of fever, or of keeping track of the height and weight of an infant to check growth, or getting TSH levels on people with suspected thyroid problems. Why, then, are there a multitude of articles addressing the problems of trying to test for validity? There are two answers to this question: the nature of *what* is being measured; and the *relationship* of that variable to its purported cause.

Many variables measured in the health sciences are physical quantities, such as height, serum cholesterol level, or bicarbonate. As such, they are readily observable, either directly or with the correct instruments. Irrespective of who manufactured the thermometer, different nurses will get the same reading, within the limits of reliability discussed in Chapters 8 and 9. Moreover, there is little question that what is being measured is temperature; no one would state that the height of the mercury in the tube is really due to something else, like blood pressure or pH level.

The situation is different when we turn to variables like 'range of motion', 'quality of life', or 'responsibility as a physician'. As we discuss later in this chapter, the measurements of these factors are dependent upon their definitions, which may vary from one person to another, and the way they are measured. For example, some theorists hold that 'social support' can be assessed by counting the number of people a person has contact with during a fixed period of time. Other theories state that the person's perceptions of who is available in times of need are more important; while yet another school of thought is that the reciprocity of the helping relationship is crucial. Since social support is not something which can be observed and measured directly, various questionnaires have been developed to assess it, each reflecting a different underlying theory. Needless to say, each instrument yields a somewhat different result, raising the question of which, if any, gives the 'correct' answer.

The second reason why validity testing is required in some areas but not others depends on the relationship between the observation and what it reflects. Based on years of observation or our knowledge of how the body works, the validity of a test may be self-evident. For instance, since the kidneys regulate the level of creatinine in the body, it makes sense to use serum creatinine to determine the presence of renal disease. On the other hand, we do not know ahead of time whether a physiotherapist's evaluations of patients' level of functioning bear any relationship to their actual performance once they are discharged from hospital. Similarly, we may hypothesize that students who have spent time doing volunteer work for service agencies will make better physicians or nurses. However, since our knowledge of the determinants of human behaviour is far from perfect, this prediction will have to be validated against actual performance.

The 'types' of validity

One of the most difficult aspects of validity testing is the terminology. Until the 1970s, almost all textbooks adopted a 'trinitarian' point of view (Landy 1986), dividing this topic into the 'three Cs' of *content* validity, *criterion* validity, and *construct* validity (terms we will discuss later). These were seen as three relatively separate attributes of a measure which had to be independently established. More recently, though, two seemingly different trends have emerged. First, a proliferation of new 'types' of validity were proposed. For example, construct validity was differentiated into various classes such as trait validity, discriminant validity, convergent validity, and so forth (see, for example, Messick 1980). At the same time, a second trend led to a reconceptualization of the process of validity testing itself and what could actually be concluded from a demonstration of validity in one form or another.

Previously, testing for validity was seen as demonstrating the psychometric properties of a *scale*. Led by Cronbach (1971), though, the focus changed to emphasize the characteristics of the *people* who are assessed. As Landy (1986) puts it, 'Validation processes are not so much directed toward the integrity of tests as they are directed toward the inferences that can be made about the attributes of the people who have produced those test scores' (p. 1186). In other words, validating a scale is really a process whereby we determine the degree of confidence we can place on inferences we make about people based on their scores from that scale.

Seen from this perspective, the two trends are actually just different aspects of the same thing. Validation is a process of *hypothesis testing*: 'Someone who scores high on this measure will also do well in situation A, perform poorly on test B, and will differ from those who score low on the scale on traits C and D'. So, rather than being constrained by the trinitarian Cs mentioned above, scale constructors are limited only by their imagination in devising experiments to test their hypotheses. In the past, students (and their teachers) have spent much time arguing whether a specific study demonstrated, for example, criterion or construct validity. Now, the important questions are, 'Does the hypothesis of this validation study make sense in light of what the scale is designed to measure', and 'Do the results of this study allow us to draw the inferences that we wish to make?'

Unfortunately, this creates difficulties for writers of textbooks. From the new perspective, a chapter on validity would focus primarily on the logic and methodology of hypothesis testing. The student, though, will continue to encounter terms like 'construct validity' and 'criterion validity' in his or her readings for some time to come. We have chosen here to take the middle ground; to organize the chapter around the traditional headings, but at the same time to emphasize that rather than being disparate attributes, the various 'types' of validity are all addressing the same issue of the degree of confidence we can place in the inferences we draw from scores on scales.

Content validity

We mentioned content validity previously within the context of issues surrounding item construction (Chapter 3). Here, let us briefly touch on it again from our new vantage point. When we conclude that a student has 'passed' a test in, say, respirology, or that an arthritic patient has a grip strength of only 10 kg, we are making the assumption that the measures comprise representative samples of the disorders, behaviours, attitudes, or knowledge that we want to assess. That is, we do not too much care if the student knows the specific bits of information tapped by the examination, or how much the patient can squeeze a dynamometer. Going back to what validity testing is all about, our aim is *inferential*; a person who does well on the exam can be expected to know more about lungs than a student who does poorly, and a patient who has a weaker grip has more severe arthritis than someone who can exert more pressure.

A measure that includes a more representative sample of the target behaviour lends itself to more accurate inferences; that is, inferences which hold true under a wider range of circumstances. If there are important aspects of the outcome that are missed by the scales, then we are likely to make some inferences which will prove to be wrong; our *inferences* (not the instruments) are invalid. For example, if there was nothing on the respirology examination regarding oxygen exchange, then it is quite possible that a high scorer on the test may *not* know more about this topic than a student with a lower score. Similarly, grip strength has relatively poor content validity; as such, it does not allow us to make accurate inferences about other attributes of the rheumatoid patient, such as erythrocyte sedimentation rate, joint count, or morning stiffness, except insofar as these indices are correlated with grip strength.

Thus, the higher the content validity of a measure, the broader are the inferences that we can validly draw about the person under a variety of conditions and in different situations.

We discussed in previous chapters that reliability places an upper limit on validity, so that the higher the reliability, the higher the maximum possible validity (more formally, the maximum validity of a test is the square root of reliability coefficient). There is one notable exception to this general rule: the relationship between internal consistency (an index of reliability) and content validity. If we are tapping a behaviour, disorder, or trait that is relatively heterogeneous, like rheumatoid arthritis, then it is quite conceivable that the scale will have low internal consistency; not all patients with a high joint count have a high sedimentation rates or morning stiffness. We could increase the internal consistency of the index by eliminating items which are not highly correlated with each other or the total score. If we did this, though, we would end up with an index tapping only one aspect of arthritis—stiffness, for example—and which therefore has very low content validity. Under such circumstances, it is better to sacrifice internal consistency for content validity. The ultimate aim of the scale is inferential, which depends more on content validity than internal consistency.

Criterion validity

The traditional definition of criterion validity is the correlation of a scale with some other measure of the trait or disorder under study, ideally, a 'gold standard' which has been used and accepted in the field. Criterion validity is usually divided into two types: *concurrent* validity and *predictive* validity. With concurrent validity, we correlate the new scale with the criterion measure, both of which are given at the same time. For example, we could administer a new scale for depression and the *Beck Depression Inventory* (an accepted measure of depression) during the same interview, or within a short time of each other. In predictive validity, the criterion will not be available until some time in the future. The major areas where this latter form of criterion validity is used are in college admission tests, where the ultimate outcome is the person's performance on graduation four years hence; or diagnostic tests, where we must await the

outcome of an autopsy or the further progression of the disease to confirm or dis-
confirm our predictions.

A major question is why, if a good criterion measure already exists, are we
going through the often laborious process of developing a new instrument?
Leaving aside the unworthy (if prevalent) reasons of trying to cash in on a lucra-
tive market, or having an instrument with one's name as part of the title, there
are a number of valid reasons. The existing test can be expensive, invasive,
dangerous, or time-consuming; or the outcome may not be known until it is too
late. The first four reasons are the usual rationales for scales which require concurrent validation, and the last reason for those which need predictive validity.
On the basis of these reasons for developing new tests, Messick (1980) has proposed using the terms *diagnostic utility* or *substitutability* for concurrent validity,
and *predictive utility* for predictive validity; while they are not yet widely used,
these are far more descriptive terms for the rationales underlying criterion validity testing.

As an example of the use of concurrent validity, let us look at the usual standard test for tuberculosis, the chest X-ray. While it is still used as the definitive
criterion, it suffers from a number of drawbacks which make it a less than ideal
test, especially for routine screening. It is somewhat invasive—exposing the
patient to low levels of ionizing radiation, and expensive—requiring a costly
machine, film, a trained technician, and a radiologist to interpret the results. For
these reasons, it would be desirable to develop a cheaper and less risky test for
screening purposes. This new tool would then be compared, in a concurrent validation study, to the chest X-ray.

Within the realm of predictive validity, we would like to know *before* students
are admitted to graduate or professional school whether or not they will graduate four years later, rather than having to incur the expense of the training and
possibly denying admission to someone who will do well. So, administering our
scale prior to admission, we would determine how well it predicts graduate
status or performance on a licensing examination.

Let us go through the usual procedures for establishing these two forms of validity and their rationales. As we have mentioned, the most commonly used
design for concurrent validity is to administer the new scale and the standard at
the same time. Staying with the example of a new test for TB, we would give
both the Mantoux test (assuming it is the one being validated) and the X-ray to a
large group of people. Since the outcome is dichotomous (the person either has
or does not have abnormalities on the X-ray consistent with TB), we would draw
up a fourfold table, as in Table 10.1.

We could analyse the results using either the indices of sensitivity and specificity, or some measure of correlation which can be derived from a 2×2 table,
such as the phi coefficient (ϕ). This coefficient is related to χ^2 by the formula

$$\phi = \sqrt{\frac{\chi^2}{N}} \, ,$$

Table 10.1 *Fourfold table to evaluate criterion validity for scales with dichotomous outcomes*

X-ray results

	TB	No TB
Mantoux test — TB	a	b
No TB	c	d

or can be calculated from Table 10.1 using the equation

$$\phi = \frac{|\ BC - AD\ |}{\sqrt{[(A + B)\ (C + D)\ (A + C)\ (B + D)]}}.$$

If our measures were continuous, as would be found if we were validating a new measure of depression against the *Beck Depression Inventory* or *CES-D* (another accepted index of depression), we would use a Pearson correlation coefficient. In either case, we would be looking for a strong association between our new measure and the already existing one. This would indicate that a person who has a high score or comes out 'diseased' on the new test would be expected to have a high score (or have been labelled as diseased) on the more established instrument.

In assessing predictive validity, the person is given the new measure at Time 1, and then the standard some time later, at Time 2. Again, we would use a four-fold table to evaluate a scale with a dichotomous outcome, and a correlational measure if the outcome were continuous. However, there is one additional point which appears obvious, but is often overlooked; *no decision can be made based on the new instrument.* For example, if we were trying to establish the validity of an autobiographical letter as a criterion for admission to medical or nursing school, we would have all applicants write these missives. Then, no matter how good we felt this measure was, we would immediately put the evaluations of the letters in a safe place, without looking at them, and base our decisions on other criteria. Only after the students had or had not graduated would we take out the scores, and compare them with actual performance.

What would happen if we violated this proscription, and used the letters to help us decide who should be admitted? We would be able to determine what proportion of students who wrote excellent letters graduated four years later (cell A in Table 10.1) and what proportion failed (cell B). However, we would *not* be able to state what proportion of those who wrote 'poor' letters would have gone on to pass with flying colours (cell C), nor how good letters are in detecting people who will fail (cell D): they would never be given the chance. In this case, the sample has been *truncated* on the basis of our new test and, as we will describe later in more detail, the correlation between our new test and the standard will be reduced, perhaps significantly.

A somewhat different situation can also occur with diagnostic tests. If the final diagnosis (the gold standard) were predicated in part on the results of our new instrument, then we have artificially built in a high correlation between the two; we are correlating the new measure with an outcome based on it. For example, in the process of validating two-dimensional echo-cardiography for diagnosing mitral valve prolapse (MVP), we would use the clinician's judgement of the presence or absence of MVP as the criterion. However, the clinician may know the results of the echo tests, and temper his diagnosis in light of them. This differs from our previous example in that we have not truncated our sample; rather, we are indirectly using the results of our new scale in both the predictor and the outcome. The technical term for this is *criterion contamination*.

In summary, then, criterion validity assesses how a person who scores at a certain level on our new scale does on some criterion measure. The usual experimental design is a correlational one; both measures are taken on a series of individuals. In the case of concurrent validity, the two results are gathered close together in time. In predictive validity, the results from the criterion measure are usually not known for some time, which can be between a few days to a few years later.

Construct validity

What is construct validity?

Attributes such as height or weight are readily observable, or can be 'operationally defined'; that is, defined by the way they are measured. Systolic blood pressure, for example, is the amount of pressure, measured in millimeters of mercury, at the moment of ventricular systole. Once we move away from the realm of physical attributes into more 'psychological' ones like anxiety, intelligence, or pain, however, we begin dealing with more abstract variables, ones that cannot be directly observed. We cannot 'see' anxiety; all we can observe are behaviours which, according to our theory of anxiety, are the results of it. We would attribute the sweaty palms, tachycardia, pacing back and forth, and difficulty in concentrating experienced by a student just prior to writing an exam, to his or her anxiety. Similarly, we may have two patients who, to all intents and purposes, have the same degree of angina. One patient has quit his job and spends most of the day sitting in a chair; the other continues working and is determined to 'fight it'. We may explain these differences in terms of such attitudes as 'motivation', 'illness behaviour', or the 'sick role model'. Again, these factors are not seen directly, only their hypothesized manifestations in terms of the patients' observable behaviours.

These proposed underlying factors are referred to as *hypothetical constructs*, or, more simply as *constructs*. A construct can be thought of as a 'mini-theory' to explain the relationships among various behaviours or attitudes. Many constructs arose from larger theories or clinical observations, before there were any ways of objectively measuring their effects. This would include terms like 'anxiety' or 'repression', derived from psychoanalytic theory; or 'sick role behaviour', which was based mainly on sociological theorizing. Other concepts, like the difference between 'fluid' and 'crystallized' intelligence (Cattell 1963), were proposed to explain observed correlations among variables which were already measured with a high degree of reliability.

It is fair to say that most psychological instruments and many measures of health are designed to tap some aspect of a hypothetical construct. There are two reasons for wanting to develop such an instrument: the construct is a new one, and no scale exists which measures it; or we are dissatisfied with the existing tools, and feel that they omit some key aspect of the construct. Note that we are doing more than replacing one tool with a shorter, cheaper, or less invasive one, which is the rationale for criterion validity. Rather, we are using the underlying theory to help us develop a new or better instrument, where 'better' means able to explain a broader range of findings, explain them in a more parsimonious manner, or make more accurate predictions about a person's behaviour.

Establishing construct validity

As an example, consider the quest to develop a short checklist or scale to identify patients with irritable bowel syndrome (IBS). First, though, we should address the issue of why we consider IBS to be a construct rather than a disease like ulcers or amoebic dysentery. The central issue is that we cannot (at least not yet) definitively prove that a person has IBS; it is diagnosed by excluding other possible causes of the patient's symptoms. There is no X-ray or laboratory test to which we can point and say, 'Yes, that person has IBS'. Moreover, there is no known pathogen which produces the constellation of symptoms. We tie them together conceptually by postulating an underlying disorder which cannot be measured directly, in much the same way that we say a large vocabulary, a breadth of knowledge, and skill at problem-solving are all outward manifestations of a postulated but unseen concept we label 'intelligence'. Many of what physicians call 'syndromes' would be called 'hypothetical constructs' by psychologists and test developers. Indeed, even some 'diseases' like schizophrenia, Alzheimer's, or systemic lupus erythematosus, are closer to constructs than actual entities, since their diagnosis is based on constellations of symptoms, and there are no unequivocal diagnostic tests which can be used with living patients. This is more than just semantics, though. It implies that tests for diagnosing or measuring syndromes should be constructed in an analogous manner to those for more 'psychological' attributes.

The first indices developed for assessing IBS consisted, in the main, of two parts: exclusion of other diseases, and the presence of some physical signs and symptoms like pain in the lower left quadrant and diarrhoea without pain. These scales proved to be inadequate, as many patients 'diagnosed' by them were later discovered to have stomach cancer or other diseases, and patients who were missed were, a few years later, indistinguishable from IBS patients. Thus, new scales were developed which added other—primarily demographic and person-ality—factors, predicated on a broader view (a revised construct) of IBS, as a disorder marked by specific demography and a unique psychological config-uration, in addition to the physical symptoms. The problem the test developers now faced was how to demonstrate that the new index was better than the older ones.

To address this problem, let us go back to what we mean by a 'valid' scale: it is one that allows us to make accurate inferences about a person. These inferences are derived from the construct, and are of the form; 'Based on my theory of con-struct X, people who score high on a test of X differ from people who score low on it in terms of attributes A, B, and C', where A, B, and C can be other instru-ments, behaviours, diagnoses, and so on. In this particular case, we would say, 'Based on my concept of IBS, high scorers on the index should (a) have symp-toms which will not clear with conventional therapy, and (b) have a lower preva-lence of organic bowel disease on autopsy'.

Since we are testing constructs, this form of testing is called *construct valida-tion*. Methodologically, it differs from the types of validity testing we discussed previously in a number of important ways. First, content and criterion validity can often be established with one or two studies. However, we are often able to make many different predictions based on our theory or construct. For example, if we were validating a new scale of anxiety, just a few of the many hypotheses we can derive would be, 'Anxious people would have more rapid heart rates dur-ing an exam than low anxious ones'; 'Anxious people should do better on simple tasks than non-anxious subjects, but poorer than them on complex tasks'; or 'If I artificially induce anxiety with some experimental manoeuvre, then the subjects should score higher on my test'.

Thus, there is no one single experiment which can unequivocally 'prove' a construct. Construct validation is an on-going process, of learning more about the construct, making new predictions, and then testing them. Albert Einstein once said that there have been hundreds of experiments supporting his theory of relativity, but it would take only one non-confirmatory study to disprove it. So it is with construct validation; each supportive study serves only to strengthen what Cronbach and Meehl (1955) call the 'nomological network' of the interlocking predictions of a theory, but a single, well-designed experiment with negative findings can call into question the entire construct.

A second major difference between construct validity and the other types is that, with the former, we are assessing both the theory and the measure at the same time. Returning to our example of a better index for IBS, one prediction was that patients who have a high score would not respond to conventional therapy. Assume that we gave the index to a sample of patients presenting at a gastrointestinal (GI) clinic, and gave them all regular treatment. (Remember, we cannot base any decisions on the results of a scale we are validating; this would lead to criterion contamination.) If it turned out that our prediction were confirmed, then it would lend credence to both our concept of IBS and the index we developed to measure it. However, if high-scoring subjects responded to treatment in about the same proportion as low scorers, then the problem could be that:

- our instrument is good, but the theory is wrong,
- the theory is fine, but our index cannot discriminate between IBS patients and those with other GI problems, or
- both the theory is wrong and our scale is useless.

Moreover, we would have no way of knowing which of these situations obtains until we do more studies.

A further complication enters the picture when we use an experimental study to validate the scale. Using the example of a new measure of anxiety, one prediction was that if we artificially induce anxiety, as in threatening the subject with an electric shock if he or she performs poorly on some task, then we should see an increase in scores on the index. If the scores do not go up, then the problem could be in either of the areas already mentioned—the theory and the measure—plus one other; both the theory and the scale are fine, but the experiment did not induce anxiety, as we had hoped it would. Again, any combination of these problems could be working: the measure is valid and the experiment worked, but the theory is wrong; the theory is right and the experiment went the way we planned, but the index is not measuring anxiety; and so forth.

We said that construct validity differs from content and criterion validity methodologically. At the risk of being repetitive, we should emphasize that construct validation does not *conceptually* differ from the other types. To quote Guion (1977), '*All* validity is at its base some form of construct validity . . . . It *is* the basic meaning of validity' (p. 410).

It should not be surprising that given the greater complexity and breadth of questions asked with construct validity as compared with the other types of validity, there are many more ways of establishing it. In the next section, we will discuss only a few of these methods: extreme groups, convergent and discriminant validity, and the multitrait—multimethod matrix. Many other experimental and quasi-experimental approaches exist; the interested reader should consult some of the references listed in Appendix A.

Extreme groups
Perhaps the easiest experiment to conceive of in assessing the validity of a scale is to give it to two groups; one of which has the trait or behaviour, and the other

which does not. The former group should score significantly higher (or lower, depending on how the items are scored) on the new instrument. This is sometimes called construct validation by *extreme groups*. We can use the attempt to develop a better scale for IBS as an example. Using their best tools, experienced clinicians would divide a group of patients presenting to a GI clinic into two subgroups: those whom they feel have IBS and those who have some other bowel disorder. To make the process of scale development easier, all patients with equivocal diagnoses would be eliminated in this type of study.

Although this type of design appears quite straightforward, it has buried within it two methodological problems. The first difficulty with the method is that if we are trying to develop a new or better tool, how can we select the extreme groups? To be able to do so would imply that there is already an instrument in existence which meets our needs. There is no ready solution to this problem. In practice, the groups are selected using the best *available* tool, even if it is the relatively crude criterion of 'expert judgement', or a scale that almost captures what our new scale is designed to tap. We can then use what Cronbach and Meehl (1955) call 'bootstrapping'. If the new scale allows us to make more accurate predictions, or explain more findings, or achieve better inter-observer agreement, then it can replace the original criterion. In turn, then, it can be used as the gold standard against which a newer or revised version can be validated; hence 'pulling ourselves up by the bootstraps'.

The second methodological problem is one that occurs with diagnostic tests, and which is often overlooked in the pressure to publish; the extreme group design may be a necessary step, but it is by no means sufficient. That is, it is minimally necessary for our new scale to be able to differentiate between those people who obviously have the disorder or trait in question and those who do not; if the scale cannot do this, it is probably useless in all other regards. However, the question must be asked, 'Is this the way the instrument will be used in practice?' If we are trying to develop a new diagnostic tool, the answer most often is 'no'. We likely would not need a new test to separate out the obvious cases from the obvious non-cases. Especially in a tertiary care setting, the people who are sent are in the middle range; they *may* have the disorder, but then again there are some doubts. If it is with this group that the instrument will be used, then the ultimate test of its usefulness is in making these much finer discriminations.

For example, many instruments have been designed to detect the presence of organic brain syndrome (OBS). As a first step, we would try out such a tool on one group of patients with confirmed brain damage and on another where there is no evidence of any pathology. These two groups should be clearly distinguishable on the new test. However, such patients are rarely referred for neuropsychological assessment, since their diagnoses (or lack thereof) are readily apparent based on other criteria. The next step, then, would be to try this instrument on the types of patients who *would* be sent for assessment, where the differential diagnosis is between OBS and depression, a difficult discrimination to make. These groups would be formed based on the best guess of a psychiatrist, perhaps augmented by some other tests of OBS, ones we are trying to replace.

Convergent and discriminant validity

Assessing the validity by using extreme groups is closely related to *convergent validity*; seeing how closely the new scale is related to other variables and other measures of the same construct to which it should be related. For example, if our theory states that anxious people are supposed to be more aware of autonomic nervous system (ANS) activity than non-anxious people, then scores on the new index of anxiety should correlate with scores on a measure of autonomic awareness. Again, if the scores do *not* correlate, then the problem can be our new scale, the measure of autonomic sensitivity, or our theory. On the other hand, we do not want the scales to be too highly correlated; this would indicate that they are measuring the same thing, that the new one is nothing more than a different measure of autonomic awareness. How high is 'too high?' As usual, it all depends. If ANS sensitivity is, by our theory, a major component of anxiety, then the correlation should be relatively robust; if it is only one of many components of anxiety, then the correlation should be lower.

The other aspect of convergent validity is that the new index of anxiety should correlate with other measures of this construct. Again, while the correlation should be high, it should not be overly high if we believe that our new anxiety scale covers components of this trait not tapped by the existing ones.

Not only should our construct correlate with related variables, it should *not* correlate with dissimilar, unrelated ones; what we refer to as *discriminant validity*. If our theory states that anxiety is independent of intelligence, then we should not find a strong correlation between the two. Finding one may indicate, for example, that the wording of our instrument is so difficult that intelligence is playing a role in simply understanding the items. Of course, the other reasons may also apply; our scale, the intelligence test, or the construct may be faulty.

The multitrait–multimethod matrix

A powerful technique for looking at convergent and discriminant validity simultaneously is called the *multitrait–multimethod* matrix, or MTMM (Campbell and Fiske 1959). Two or more different, usually unrelated, traits are each measured by two or more methods at the same time. The two traits, for instance, can be 'self-directed learning' and 'knowledge' (assuming that they are relatively unrelated), each assessed by a rater and a written exam. This leads to a matrix of 10 correlations, as shown with fictitious data in Table 10.2.

The numbers in parentheses (0.53, 0.79, etc.) along the main diagonal are the reliabilities of the four instruments. The two italicized figures, *0.42* and *0.49*, are the 'homotrait–heteromethod' correlations: the same trait (e.g. knowledge) measured in different ways. Those in curly brackets {0.18} and {0.23} are 'heterotrait–homomethod' correlations: different traits assessed by the same

Table 10.2   *A fictitious multitrait-multimethod matrix*

		Self-directed learning		Knowledge	
		Rater	Exam	Rater	Exam
Self-directed learning	Rater	(0.53)			
	Exam	*0.42*	(0.79)		
Knowledge	Rater	{0.18}	[0.17]	(0.58)	
	Exam	[0.15]	{0.23}	*0.49*	(0.88)

method. Finally, the heterotrait–heteromethod correlations are in square brackets [0.17] and [0.15]: different traits measured with different methods.

Ideally, the highest correlations should be the reliabilities of the individual measures; an examination of 'knowledge' given on two occasions should yield higher correlations than examinations of different traits or two different ways of tapping knowledge. Similarly, the lowest correlations should be the heterotrait—heteromethod ones; different traits measured by different methods should not be related.

Convergent validity is reflected in the homotrait–heteromethod correlations; different measures of the same trait should correlate with each other. In this example, the results of the written exam should correlate with scores given by the rater for 'knowledge', and similarly for the two assessments of 'self-directed learning'. Conversely, discriminant validity is shown by low correlations when the same method (e.g. the written exam) is applied to different traits—the heterotrait—homomethod coefficients. If they are as high or higher than the homotrait–heteromethod correlations, this would show that the *method* of measurement was more important than *what* was being measured. This is obviously an undesirable property, since the manner of assessing various attributes should be secondary to the relationship that should exist between various ways of tapping into the same trait.

It is often difficult to do studies appropriate for the MTMM approach because of the time required on the subjects' part, as well the problem of finding different methods of assessing the same trait. When these studies can be done, though, they can address a number of validity issues simultaneously.

Summary

Unlike criterion validity, then, there is no one experimental design or statistic which is common to construct validational studies. If one of the hypotheses is that our new measure of a construct is related to other indices of that construct or that the construct should be associated with other constructs, then the study is usually correlational in nature; our new scale and another one (of the same or a related construct) are given to the subjects. If one hypothesis is that some naturally occurring group has 'more' of the construct than another group, then we can simply give our new instrument to both groups, and look for differences between the two means. Still another hypothesis may be that if we give some experimental or therapeutic intervention, it will affect the construct and the measure of it; transcutaneous stimulation should reduce pain, while intense radiant heat should increase it. In this instance, our study could be a before–after trial or, more powerfully, a true experiment whereby one group receives the intervention and the other does not. If our construct is correct, and the manoeuvre worked, and our scale is valid, then we should see differences between the groups.

In summary, it is obviously necessary to conduct validational studies for each new instrument we develop. However, when the scale is one measuring a hypothetical construct, the task is an on-going one. New hypotheses derived from the construct require new studies. Similarly, if we want to use the measure with groups it was not initially validated on, we must first demonstrate that the inferences we make for them are as valid as for the original population. Finally, modifications of existing scales often require new validity studies. For example, if we wanted to use the D scale of the MMPI as an index of depression, we cannot assume that it is as valid when used in isolation as when the items are imbedded amongst 500 other, unrelated ones. It is possible that the mere fact of presenting them together gives the patient a different orientation and viewpoint.

Biases in validity assessment

Restriction in range

We mentioned in Chapter 8 that an unacceptable way of seeming to increase the reliability of a measure is to give it to a more heterogeneous group than the one it is designed for. In this section, we return to this point from a different perspective; how the range of scores affects the validity of the scale. There are actually three ways this can occur:

* the predictor variable (usually our new measure) is restricted;
* the criterion is restricted; and
* a third variable, correlated with both the predictor and criterion variables, is used to select the group which will be given the predictor and criterion variables.

As an example, assume that we have read about a new assay for serum monoamine oxidase (MAO) which is highly correlated with scores on a depression inventory. In the original (fictitious) article, a correlation of 0.80 was

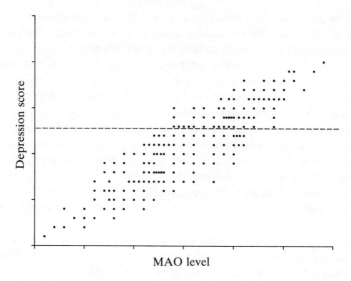

Fig. 10.1. Scatterplot showing the relationship between two variables.

found in a large community-based sample. Such an assay would be extremely useful in a hospital setting, where difficulty with the English language and the various biases (e.g. faking good or bad) are often problems with self-adminis-tered scales. We replicate the study on our in-patient psychiatry ward, but find a disappointingly low correlation of only 0.37. Should we be surprised?

Based on our discussion of restriction of range, the answer is 'no'. We can illustrate this effect pictorially by drawing a scatter diagram of the two variables in the original study as in Figure 10.1.

As a brief reminder, a scatterplot is made by placing a dot at the intersection of a person's scores on the two variables. Alternatively, an ellipse can be drawn so that it includes (usually) 95 per cent of the people. The more elliptical the swarm of points or the ellipse, the stronger the correlation; the more circular the ellipse, the lower the association, with the extreme being a circle reflecting a total lack of any relationship. This scatterplot is fairly thin, as would be expected with a correlation of 0.80.

In our study, all of the subjects were hospitalized depressives, so their scores on the depression inventory are expected to be higher than those in a community sample, falling above the line in Figure 10.1. As can be seen, the portion of the ellipse falling above the line is more circular than the whole scatterplot, indicat-ing that for this more restricted sample, the correlation between the two vari-ables is considerably lower.

Using some equations developed by Thorndike (1949), we can predict how much the validity coefficient will be affected by selecting more restricted groups based on the criterion (X), the predictor (Y), or some other variable (Z). The first situation would apply if patients were hospitalized only if their scores on the depression inventory exceeded a certain level. This would be the case if high scores on the scale were one of the criteria for admission, and would be analogous to validating a new TB test only on patients who have lesions on an X-ray. In this case, the validity of the predictor would be:

$$r' = \frac{r \, (s'_x/s_x)}{\sqrt{[1 - r^2 + r^2 \, (s'^2_x/s^2_x)]}}$$

where r' is the restricted validity coefficient, r is the validity coefficient in the unrestricted sample, s'_x is the SD of the criterion for the restricted sample, and s_x is the SD of the criterion for the unrestricted sample.

If the standard deviation in the unrestricted sample was 10, and it was reduced to 3 in the restricted sample, we would get:

$$\frac{0.80 \times (3/10)}{\sqrt{[1 - 0.64 + 0.64 \times (9/100)]}} = 0.37.$$

By the same token, we can work backwards by transforming this formula. If we did a study on a sample that was in some way constrained on the criterion variable, we could figure out what the validity coefficient would be if the full range of the variable were available. In this case, the formula would be:

$$r = \frac{r' \, (s_x/s'_x)}{\sqrt{[1 - r'^2 + r'^2 \, (s^2_x/s'^2_x)]}}$$

where the terms have the same meaning as above.

The second case occurs when the group is selected on the basis of the *predictor* variable (Y); using the same example, only patients with increased MAO levels are included. This is the situation that obtains with criterion contamination; students are selected based on their scores on the admission test, which is actually being evaluated to see if it is a valid predictor. The formulae are the same, except that s'_y is substituted for s'_x, and s_y for s_x.

The last case is where the subjects are selected on the basis of some other variable (Z), which is correlated with both X and Y. Using our original example, this is the most realistic condition, since patients are admitted because of the severity of their symptomatology, which is related to both MAO level and scores on the depression inventory. The question can again be asked in two ways: (1) if we know the results from an (unrestricted) community-based study, what would the correlation be in our (more restricted) hospital environment; or (2), if we correlated X and Y in our restricted sample, what would the correlation be in an unrestricted one? Since an additional variable is involved (Z, the severity of depression), more information needs to be known: (1) the correlation of X and Y in the unrestricted sample; (2) the correlations of X with Z and Y with Z in this sample; and (3) the standard deviation of Z in the restricted and unrestricted samples. As these data are rarely known, the equation is mainly of academic interest. For those who are interested, a thorough treatment of this topic can be found in Ghiselli (1964).

Unreliability of the criterion

One pervasive problem in validation occurs when we correlate our new scale with a gold standard. Quite frequently, though, the criterion is not as good as this term suggests, since it is unreliable in its own right. Thus, the validity coefficient may be attenuated since, even if the predictor (Y) were excellent, it is predicting to an unreliable criterion (X). We can estimate what the validity coefficient would be if the criterion were perfectly reliable by using the formula:

$$r_{XY}' = \frac{r_{XY}}{\sqrt{(r_{XX})}}$$

where r_{XY}' is the estimated correlation with a perfectly reliable criterion, r_{XY} is the actual correlation between tests X and Y, and r_{XX} is the reliability coefficient of the criterion (test X).

If we assume that the criterion is perfectly reliable, and we want to see how much the correlation *could* improve if the new test were perfectly reliable, we would simply substitute r_{YY} for r_{XX} under the radical:

$$r_{XY}' = \frac{r_{XY}}{\sqrt{(r_{YY})}}.$$

A more general (and realistic) case assumes that both scales are unreliable, and we want to see what the correlation would be if both were perfectly reliable. The equation now reads:

$$r_{XY}' = \frac{r_{XY}}{\sqrt{(r_{XX}\,r_{YY})}}.$$

The most general (and realistic) case is that perfect reliability never exists, in either the new instrument or in the criterion. However, it may be possible to improve the reliability of one or both, and we would want to know what the correlation between the two indices would be, given these improved (albeit not perfect) reliabilities. In this case, we would use the equation:

$$r_{XY}' = \frac{r_{XY}\,\sqrt{(r_{XX}'\,r_{YY}')}}{\sqrt{(r_{XX}\,r_{YY})}}$$

where r_{XX}' and r_{YY}' are the changed reliabilities for the two variables (somewhere between their actual reliabilities and 1.0).

These equations have two possible uses. First, they tell us how much the validity would increase if we were able to increase the reliabilities of the instruments. If the increase is only marginal, then the investment of time and perhaps money needed to improve the psychometric properties may not be worth it; whereas a large potential increase may signal that it could be worthwhile making the investment. The second useful function is in the area of theory development. If our theory tells us that variable A should correlate strongly with variable B, then correcting for unreliability of the measures gives us an indication of the true validity of the instrument, and hence of our construct. A low, uncorrected validity estimate may incorrectly lead us to discard the theory, when in fact it may be correct, and the problem is with the scales.

By the same token, it is important to remember that these corrections for attenuation tells us what the validity *can be* if we could improve the reliability of the criterion and the new instrument, not what the validity *actually is* in real life. It is worth quoting Guion (1965) in this regard: 'The effect of a possible correction for attenuation should never be a consideration when one is deciding how to evaluate a measure as it exists' (p. 32).

Changes in the sample

Life would be simple if we could establish the validity of a measure once by conducting a series of studies, and then assume that we could use that instrument under a range of circumstances and with a variety of people. Unfortunately, this is not the case. Estimates of validity, like those of reliability, are dependent upon the nature of the people being measured and, to a greater or lesser degree, the circumstances under which they are being assessed. A tool which can accurately measure the activities of daily living among cancer patients may be quite useless when used in respirology; and one that has proven valid in distinguishing OBS from depressed patients may not discriminate between OBS patients and schizophrenics. Every time a scale is used in a new context, or with a different group of people, it is necessary to re-establish its psychometric properties.

Summary

Validity is a process of determining what, if anything, we are measuring with our scale; that is, can we make valid statements about a person based on his or her score on the index. *Concurrent* validity is most often used when we are trying to replace one tool with a simpler, cheaper, or less invasive one. We generally use another form of criterion validation, called *predictive* validity, in developing instruments that allow us to get answers earlier than current instruments allow. *Construct validity* refers to a wide range of approaches which are used when what we are trying to measure is a 'hypothetical construct,' like anxiety or some syndromes, rather than something which can be readily observed.

References

Campbell, D. T. and Fiske, D. W. (1959). Convergent and discriminant validation by the multitrait-multimethod matrix. *Psychological Bulletin*, **56**, 81–105.
Cattell, R. B. (1963). Theory of fluid and crystallized intelligence: Critical experiment. *British Journal of Educational Psychology*, **54**, 1–22.

Cronbach, L. J. (1971). Test validation. In *Educational measurement* (ed. R. L. Thorndike), pp. 221–37. American Council on Education, Washington DC.

Cronbach, L. J. and Meehl, P. E. (1955) Construct validity in psychological tests. *Psychological Bulletin*, **52**, 281–302.

Ghiselli, E. E. (1964). *Theory of psychological measurement*. McGraw-Hill, New York.

Guion, R. M. (1965). *Personnel testing*. McGraw-Hill, New York.

Guion, R. M. (1977). Content validity: Three years of talk—what's the action? *Public Personnel Management*, **6**, 407–14.

Landy, F. J. (1986). Stamp collecting versus science. *American Psychologist*, **41**, 1183–92.

Messick, S. (1980). Test validity and the ethics of assessment. *American Psychologist*, **35**, 1012–27.

Thorndike, R. L. (1949). *Personnel selection: Test and measurement techniques*. Wiley, New York.

11

Measuring change

Introduction

The measurement of change has been a topic of considerable confusion in the medical literature. As clinicians and researchers, we view that the ultimate goal of most treatment—medical, surgical, psychosocial, or educational—is to induce change in the patient's or student's status. It would appear to follow that the measurement of change in patients' health state or in a student's level of understanding is an appropriate goal of research. A number of recent articles (Guyatt et al. 1987; MacKenzie et al. 1986) have advocated this position, both on the grounds that the measurement of change in patient's condition is the goal of clinical care and should be addressed by research methods, and on the methodological basis that instruments which are responsive to changes in health status are more sensitive measures of the effects of clinical interventions than those which simply assess health status after an intervention.

However, this opinion is by no means unanimous. Several authors in education and psychology have taken stands against the use of difference scores (Cronbach and Furby 1970; Burckhardt et al. 1982). In this chapter, we explore the issues surrounding the use of change scores and show that these divergent positions are based on different views of the goals of measurement, and different assumptions regarding the methodological advantages and disadvantages of change measures.

The goal of measurement of change

In order to understand the source of the controversy in the literature, it is necessary to recognize that the measurement of change can be directed at different goals. These have been described by Linn and Slinde (1977).
1. *To measure differences between individuals in the amount of change*. Although apparently similar to the notion of reliability, the intent is to distinguish between those individuals who *change a lot* and those who *change little*. For example, if we wanted to identify individuals who were responsive to therapy (e.g. in a secondary analysis of a trial of therapy for arthritis), we would proceed by a comparison of individual differences in change scores. Much of the literature in

psychology addressing the measurement of change accepts this as the basic goal of change measurement.

2. *To identify correlates of change.* This goal really represents an elaboration of the first. If we were successful at identifying responsive sub-groups in a trial of therapy, a logical second step is to attempt to identify those factors which are associated or correlated with good response. The issues of measurement also follow from the earlier concerns: if we cannot differentiate between those who change a great deal and those who change little, the resulting restriction in range will attenuate any attempt to find correlates.

3. *To infer treatment effects from group differences.* This goal is probably the primary goal of most clinical trials. By randomly assigning individuals to treatment and control groups, measuring the health state before and after treatment, and then comparing the average change in health state in the groups, we can determine a treatment effect—individuals in a treatment group will change, on the average, more than those in a control group.

The first and last goals work against one another. To the extent that there are individual differences in response to treatment, this is an indication that the treatment had different effects on different people, and it will be more difficult to detect an overall treatment effect. However, if there are individual differences in response to treatment, then we will be able to identify responsive sub-groups and possible prognostic factors; if there are no individual differences, we will be unsuccessful in this search.

Note however, that there is no conflict in the goal of discrimination between individuals, as expressed in the reliability coefficient, and the goal of evaluation of change within individuals. It is certainly possible that there may be large and stable differences between individuals on some measure, yet all may change equally in response to treatment. If we consider the everyday example of dieting, overweight people may range from 60 kg to 150 kg; yet a conservative and successful diet would have all losing from 1 to 2 kg per week. As long as there was reasonable consistency in the amount of weight loss experienced by different individuals in the plan, it would not be difficult to demonstrate the efficacy of a treatment program which showed losses of this order, despite the large differences in individual weights. So the presence of large differences among individuals does not, of itself, preclude the demonstration of small treatment effects. Differences in *change* of different individuals *does* reduce the chance of demonstrating overall treatment effects.

Why not measure change directly?

The remainder of this chapter will address different ways to combine measures taken at various times (usually two) to best measure the amount of change in individuals or groups. This seems, on the surface, to be a complicated way to go about things. Why not simply ask people how much they have changed, which appears a much more straightforward method? Clinicians do it all the time; for example, the following seem likely ways to ask the question:

'Since I put you on the new drug at your last visit, have you got better or worse? How much?'

'Since your illness began a few months ago, have you been getting better or worse? How much?'

'Thinking back to when you first noticed this symptom, how much worse has it got?'

Although this is a time-honoured approach, there is a very good reason to avoid asking about change directly: people simply do not remember how they were at the beginning. We have already noted in Chapter 5 that 42 per cent of patients did not remember that they had been in hospital one year after the event. It seems likely that even greater bias may affect subjective assessment of change in illnesses, whose onset and course are rarely as vivid as a hospitalization. Unfortunately, however, it is not that people will not answer the question; few will hesitate to voice an opinion. But careful research has demonstrated that, although it is relatively easy to elicit a response, the validity of the response is debatable.

Ross (1989) theorized, and then proved, that the response to a direct question about change proceeds in two discrete, but frequently unaware, steps. First, people note their present status on the attribute in question, for example 'How do I feel today?'. They then invoke an 'implicit theory' about how they are likely to have changed from the previous occasion to the present, such as 'Well, I think the drug has worked a bit better than the one the doctor had me on before'. On the basis of these two pieces of information, they then reconstruct an estimate of their previous state.

We must emphasize the word 'implicit'. As we described it, this process seems available to introspection, and hence to correction. But the nature of the process is that, like many aspects of memory, it may be unavailable to conscious introspection. But if it is unavailable to conscious thought how, then, did the researchers prove that this theory explained people's assessment of change?

As it turns out, quite simply. In a series of experiments, people were asked to rate their level on some attribute at two times directly. Then, on the second occasion, they were also asked to estimate how much they had changed since the first occasion. The approach has been applied to a wide variety of attitudes, such as estimates of attractiveness of dating partners (McFarland and Ross 1987), recall of political attitudes (Niemi *et al.* 1980), of past income (Withey 1954), and various self-improvement programs (Conway and Ross 1984). There are two general findings:

1. Estimates of the initial state from people participating in programs tend to exaggerate the effect of the program by systematically underestimating the initial state. For instance, patients in a chronic pain program retrospectively

estimated their initial pain much more severe than initially estimated (Linton and Melin 1982).

2. Retrospective estimates of initial state are typically highly correlated with the *present* state, and relatively uncorrelated with the initial state. For example, when women were asked to rate their usual degree of menstrual distress while they were menstruating, they reported systematically higher levels than did another group of women who were asked the same question during the inter-menstrual phase (McFarland *et al.* 1987). In a study of Israeli soldiers suffering from post-traumatic stress disorder (Spiro *et al.* 1989), the average correlation between subjective estimates of change and a variety of standardized symptom severity scales was +0.14 (range 0.10 to 0.27) with *pre*treatment measures; but was +0.44 (range 0.30 to 0.53) with *post*-treatment measures.

The weight of these findings suggests that direct estimation of change is fraught with bias. Some investigators have attempted to circumvent these problems by showing patients their initial estimate (for example, a pretreatment pain rating on a visual analog scale) and then asking them where they would now estimate their level to be. In our view, this does nothing to alleviate the problem. Since the evidence is that people don't really remember their initial state, such a strategy would presumably invoke a complex implicit process, where the initial rating would interact with the implicit theory and their knowledge of their present state to yield a new estimate of change. This may only compound the problem, not solve it.

It seems that the most defensible way to assess change, for estimating individual growth or treatment effects, is to directly measure the attribute at the beginning of the study period and subsequently on one or more occasions. The remainder of the chapter deals with various approaches to analysing these multiple estimates.

Measures of association—reliability, and sensitivity to change

The different goals of measurement are reflected in different coefficients, analogous to the reliability coefficient, which express the ability of an instrument to detect change within subjects or the effects of treatment. In order to clarify these distinctions, let us consider a group of six individuals who have entered into a diet plan and are weighed before treatment and again after two weeks of dieting. The data might look like Table 11.1 below.

As we discussed before, the goal of discriminating among subjects has been incorporated in the notion of *reliability*, which we discussed at length in Chapter 8, and is defined as:

$$\text{Reliability } (R) = \frac{\sigma^2_{\text{pat}}}{\sigma^2_{\text{pat}} + \sigma^2_{\text{err}}}.$$

Table 11.1 *Weight (in kg) of six patients in a diet clinic*

Patient	Before	After two weeks	Average	Change
1	150	144	147	−6
2	120	112	116	−8
3	110	108	109	−2
4	140	142	141	+2
5	138	132	135	−6
6	116	112	114	−4
Mean	129	125	127	−4.0

In the present example, the reliability focuses on the difference between patients' average weights, and σ^2_{pat} would be determined from a sum of squares calculated as:

$$SS_{pat} = (147-127)^2 + (116-127)^2 + \ldots + (114-127)^2.$$

By analogy, we can also develop a measure to describe the reproducibility of the change score, i.e. an index of the ability of the measure to discriminate between those subjects who change a great deal and those who change little.

Reliability of the change score

The assessment of the ability of an instrument to detect individual differences in change scores is appropriately labelled as the *reliability of the change score* (Lord and Novick, 1968). By analogy to the reliability coefficient, this can be expressed as:

$$\text{Reliability } (D) = \frac{\sigma^2_D}{\sigma^2_D + \sigma^2_{err(D)}}$$

where σ^2_D expresses the systematic difference between subjects in their change score, and $\sigma^2_{err(D)}$ is the error associated with this estimate. In our example, σ^2_D would be derived from a sum of squares calculated as:

$$SS_D = (-6-(-4))^2 + (-8-(-4))^2 + \ldots + (-4-)-4))^2.$$

The reliability of the change score can be shown to be related to the variance of pre-test (x) and post-test (y) scores, their reliability (R) and the correlation between pre-test and post-test (r), in the following manner:

$$\text{Reliability } (D) = \frac{\sigma_x^2 R_{xx} + \sigma_y^2 R_{yy} - 2\sigma_x\sigma_y r_{xy}}{\sigma_x^2 + \sigma_y^2 - 2\sigma_x\sigma_y r_{xy}}$$

where r_{xy} is the correlation between the pre-test and post-test. If the pre-test and post-test have the same variances, this expression reduces to:

$$\text{Reliability} = \frac{R_{xx} + R_{yy} - 2r_{xy}}{2.0 - 2r_{xy}}$$

where R_x and R_y are the reliabilities of the initial and final measurements. In our previous example, the measured reliability was 0.95. If we assume that this reliability coefficient applies equally to both pre-test and post-test, and we further assume a correlation of, say 0.80 between the two measures, then the reliability of the difference score becomes:

$$\text{Reliability } (D) = \frac{0.95 + 0.95 - 2 \times 0.80}{2.0 - 2 \times 0.80} = 0.30/0.40 = 0.75.$$

In the limiting case, it can be demonstrated that, under the circumstances where there is a perfect correlation between the pre-test and post-test scores, the reliability of the difference score is zero. Although this appears strange, it actually follows from the basic notion of discriminating between those who change a great deal and those who change little. If an experimental intervention resulted in a uniform response to treatment, all patients would improve an equal amount. As a result, the variance of the change score will be zero, since every patient's post-test score would be equal to his or her pre-test score except for a constant; no patients would have changed more or less than any other, and the reliability of the difference score would be zero.

Since a perfectly uniform response to treatment would represent an ideal state of affairs for the use of change scores to measure treatment effects, yet would yield a reliability coefficient for change scores of zero, it should not be used as an index appropriate for assessing the ability of an instrument to measure treatment effects, and some other approach must be used.

Sensitivity to change resulting from treatment effects

The preceding discussion suggests that it would be useful to devise some measure analogous to the reliability coefficient to describe an instrument's ability to detect the overall effect of treatments. This effect has been variously labelled as 'sensitivity to change' and 'responsiveness' in the literature. In contrast to the assessment of individual differences in change, there is no consensus regarding the appropriate measure of the sensitivity of a measure to the main effect of treatment. Some approaches use the magnitude of the statistical test (e.g. an *F*-ratio) to estimate sensitivity to treatment effects; other methods use various measures of the strength of effect, expressed as a ratio of the difference between groups to the variability within groups.

One approach builds on the assumptions of generalizability theory, discussed in the previous chapter. We can conceptualize the effect of treatment as a 'facet of differentiation', i.e. a variance component of interest, and all other inter-

Table 11.2 *Hypothetical data from patients at a weight loss clinic*

	Subject	Pre-test	Post-test	Difference
Diet	1	80	72	−8
	2	75	71	−4
	3	70	63	−7
	4	65	55	−10
	5	60	54	−6
Mean		70.0	63.0	−7.0
Standard deviation			8.51	2.23
	6	80	81	+1
	7	75	72	−3
Control	8	70	73	+3
	9	65	64	−1
	10	60	60	0
Mean		70.0	70.0	0.0
Standard deviation			8.21	2.23

actions as 'facets of generalization' over which we want to estimate the effect of treatment. Then we can proceed to construct a generalizability coefficient as a ratio of variances.

Returning to the example of Table 11.1, the variance component of interest in examining treatment effects is related to the average difference between post-treatment and pre-treatment scores, so is derived from a sum of squares[1] like

$$SS_{tr} = (125 - 129)^2.$$

In fact, it would be usual to attempt to evaluate treatment effects from pre-post differences in the absence of a control group, as any observed differences could be due to other explanations than the effect of treatment. More commonly, a control group would be included, and measures taken before and after treatment on both treatment and control groups. An example could be a second evaluation of diet, obtained by randomizing ten patients to treatment and control groups, then weighing each patient before and after a period of treatment. The data might resemble Table 11.2.

The appropriate statistical analysis would be to compare the difference scores of the treatment group to those of the control group using an unpaired *t*-test on the difference scores, or to conduct a repeated measures analysis of variance,

---

[1] Although the sums of squares we have calculated are useful for understanding the conceptual differences among the three measures of association, the actual sum of squares would be obtained by multiplying these calculated squared differences by the appropriate *n*'s.

Table 11.3 *Analysis of variance of diet clinic data*

Source	Sum of squares	d.f.	Mean square
Between subjects			
Treatments	61.25	1	61.25
Subjects	1040.00	8	130.00
Within subjects			
Pre-post	61.25	1	61.25
Pre-post x Treat	61.25	1	61.25
Error	200.00	8	2.50

which is mathematically equivalent, and examine the interaction between time and treatment.

The results of the analysis are shown in the ANOVA table in Table 11.3. The test of significance of the pre-post x treatment interaction involves the ratio of the mean square of the interaction, 61.25, and the mean square error, 2.50; it is expressed as an *F*-ratio:

$$F(1,8) = 61.25/2.50 = 24.50.$$

This ratio is exactly the square of an equivalent *t*-test, examining the mean difference score in the two groups.

Regardless of the statistical test employed (*t*-test of difference scores or ANOVA) in the present example, analysis of difference scores comparing treatment and control groups is the method of choice because it removes the effect of stable differences between individuals and results in a more powerful statistical test.

We can now return to the original purpose of developing a measure of sensitivity to change. As we indicated, the effect of the weight loss plan was contained in the pre-post x treatment interaction, whose variance can be estimated using the methods described in Chapters 8 and 9. In this example, the expected mean square (EMS) is equal to

$$\text{EMS} = \sigma^2_{err} + 5\sigma^2_{pre\text{-}post \text{ x } treat}.$$

Working through this equation yields an estimated variance of 11.75. The error in this estimate was equal to 2.50. These values can then be incorporated into a sensitivity to change coefficient, equal to

$$\text{Sensitivity} = \frac{\sigma^2_{change}}{\sigma^2_{change} + \sigma^2_{err}}$$

$$= \frac{11.75}{11.75 + 2.50} = 0.825.$$

The resulting coefficient expresses the proportion of the variance in the change score due to 'true', i.e. experimentally induced change. As such, it ranges from 0 to 1, and is on the same metric as the reliability coefficient. Note that the reliability coefficient and sensitivity coefficient are related but not identical. Both use the same error term, but their magnitude is related to the relative magnitude of the pre–post variance and the variance due to patients.

Difficulties with change scores in experimental designs

Potential loss of precision

Although it would appear that it is always desirable to measure change since it removes the effect of variance between patients, this is actually not the case. The calculation of a difference score is based on the difference between two quantities, the pre-test and post-test, and both are measured with some error, σ^2_{err}. If this quantity is sufficiently large relative to the variance between patients, the net result might be to introduce more, rather than less, error into the estimate of treatment effect.

The conditions under which it makes sense to measures change within patients as a measure of treatment effect can be expressed in terms of a generalizability coefficient. The use of change scores to estimate treatment main effects is only appropriate when the variance between subjects exceeds the error variance within subjects. This is equivalent to the following expression:

$$\frac{\sigma^2_{sub}}{\sigma^2_{sub} + \sigma^2_{err}} \geq 0.5.$$

Thus, one should only use change scores when the reliability of the measure exceeds 0.5. Reliability is not irrelevant or inversely related to sensitivity—*reliability is a necessary pre-condition for the appropriate application of change scores*. This analysis does not, of course, imply that measures which are reliable are, of necessity, useful for the assessment of change. Even if an instrument is reliable, it remains to be shown that differences in response to treatment can be detected before the instrument can be used for the assessment of change.

Biased measurement of treatment effects

The simple subtraction of post-treatment from pre-treatment scores to create a difference score as a measure of the overall effect of treatment assumes that the effect of treatment will be the same, except for random error, for all patients. This assumption can be shown to be false in many, if not most circumstances. One reason is that one major cause of an individual having an extreme score on pre-test is simply an accumulation of random processes; i.e. the very good scores are to some extent due to good luck, and the very bad scores are due to bad luck. To the extent that chance is operative (and any reliability coefficient less than 1 is an indication of the presence of random variation), then the very good are likely to get worse, and the very bad get better, on retest. This effect is known as 'regression to the mean'. In effect, the best line fitting post-test to pre-treatment data in the absence of treatment effects has a slope less than 1 and an intercept greater than 0. The use of change scores assumes a best fit line with a slope of 1 and intercept of 0. The consequence of regression to the mean is that the use of change or difference scores overestimates the effect of pre-test differences on post-test scores.

The solution to this problem for assessing individual change recommended by Cronbach and Furby (1970) is the use of *residualized gain scores*. Instead of subtracting pre-test from post-test, we first fit the line relating the pre-test and post-test scores using regression analysis. We then estimate the post-test score of each patient from the regression equation. The residualized gain score is the difference between the actual post-test score and the score which was predicted from the regression equation. In other words, the residualized gain score removes from consideration that portion of the gain score which was linearly predictable from the pre-test score. What remains is an indication of those individuals who changed more or less than was expected.

This operation is really designed to identify individual differences in change in an unbiased manner. Cronbach and Furby (1970) among others have commented on the use of change scores to estimate overall treatment effects, and conclude that analysis of covariance methods should be employed when the reliability is sufficiently large, and simple post-test scores otherwise.

The reason for the use of ANCOVA is again related to the phenomenon of regression to the mean. As we discussed, the change score assumes that the line relating pre-test to post-test has a slope of 1 and intercept 0, which is not the optimal line when error of measurement is present. The result is that the denominator of the statistical test of treatment effects includes variance due to lack of fit, resulting in a conservative test. Since ANCOVA fits an optimum line to the data, in general, this will result in a smaller error term and a more sensitive test of treatment effects.

Change scores and quasi-experimental designs

So far, we have addressed the use of change scores in the context of randomized trials, where the primary goal is to increase the sensitivity of statistical tests by reducing the magnitude of the error term. There is another potential application of these methods in situations such as cohort analytical studies where there are likely to be initial differences between treatment and control groups. In this situation, the change score has an apparent advantage, in that the subtraction of the initial score for each subject will have the effect of eliminating the initial differences between groups.

However, when the change score is used in a situation where there are differ-

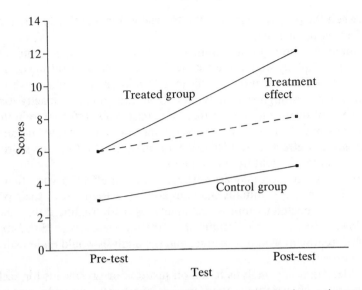

Fig. 11.1. Relation between pre-test and post-test scores in a quasi-experimental design.

ences between the two groups on the pre-test measure, as might result if subjects were not allocated at random to the two conditions, additional complications arise. These are directly related to the effect of regression to the mean, discussed in the section on residualized gain scores. In the absence of treatment effects, individuals measured with some random error will not stay the same on retest. Those who were very good will worsen, on average, and those who were very bad will improve.

Unfortunately this effect also applies to group means, which are simply the average of individual scores. In the absence of any treatment effect, the differences between groups will be reduced at the second testing, confounding any interpretation of differences between groups observed following treatment. One way around this problem is again the use of *analysis of covariance*, however this method is a refinement to the use of change scores, not a fundamentally different approach.

There are other fundamental reasons to view any attempt at post-hoc adjustment for differences between groups on pre-test, whether by difference scores, repeated measures ANOVA or ANCOVA, with considerable suspicion. Implicit in these analytical methods is a specific model of the change process which cannot be assumed to have general applicability. This is illustrated in Figure 11.1.

Any of the analytical methods assume that, in the absence of any treatment effect, the experimental and control group will grow at the same rate, so that the difference in means at the beginning would equal the difference in means at the end, and any additional difference between the two groups (shown as the difference between the post-test mean of the treated group and the dotted line) is evidence of a treatment effect.

Unfortunately, there are any number of plausible alternative models which will fit the data equally well. For example, in a rehabilitation setting or in an educational program for mentally handicapped children, individuals who are less impaired, thus score higher initially, may have the greatest capacity for change or improvement over time. Under these circumstances, referred to in the literature as a 'fan-spread' model, the observed data would be obtained in the absence of any treatment effect, and ANCOVA or analysis of difference scores would wrongly conclude a benefit from treatment.

Conversely, a situation may arise where a 'ceiling effect' occurs; that is, individuals with high scores initially may already be at the limit of their potential, thus would be expected to improve relatively less with treatment than those with initially lower scores. In this circumstance, the post-test scores in the absence of an effect of treatment would converge, and the analysis would underestimate the treatment effect.

It is evident that any analysis based on just one or two means for each group will not permit a choice among these models of growth, and additional points on the individual growth curve would be required (Rogosa *et al.* 1982). Of course, if such situations were rare, one could argue for the adequacy of change score approaches; however it is likely that situations of non-constant growth are the rule, not the exception, in health research. As Lord (1967) put it, 'there simply is no logical or statistical procedure that can be counted on to make proper allowances for uncontrolled preexisting differences between groups'.

Measuring change using multiple observations: Growth curves

In the last section, we alluded to the problems associated with inferring change from two observations. In part, these problems result from the very simple model of change which is implied by a simple pre-test–post-test approach. Change looks like a quantum process: first you're in one state, then you're in another state. Individual change obviously does not occur this way. It is a continuous process, whether we are speaking of physical change (e.g. growth or recovery from trauma), intellectual change (learning or development), or emotional change. Moreover, it is probably non-linear. Some individuals may make an initially rapid recovery from an illness and then improve slowly; some may improve gradually at first and then more rapidly; and of course some may deteriorate or fluctuate around a stable state of partial recovery.

It is evident that any reasonable attempt to characterize these individual *growth curves* will require multiple points of observation, so that a statistical curve can be fitted. While this sounds laborious, in many circumstances multiple observations are available, and only await an appropriate method for analysis. For example, many treatment programs extend across multiple visits, and frequently the clinician makes systematic observations in order to assess response to therapy and possibly adjust treatment. If multiple observations are available, it makes little sense to base an assessment of treatment effect only on assessments at the beginning and end of treatment, which would throw away a great deal of data. Even if the change is uniform and linear, so that there is no apparent advantage of assessment methods based on individual growth, the use of multiple observations amounts to an increase in sample size, with a corresponding reduction of within-subject error and an increase in statistical power.

There is a growing consensus on approaches to the appropriate analysis of data of this form, although the theory underlying such methods has a brief history, dating back only about a decade (Francis *et al.* 1991; Bryk and Raudenbush 1987; Rogosa *et al.* 1982). The basic idea common to all methods is to develop an analytical model of the relationship between individual growth and time, then estimate the parameters of the model using a variant of regression analysis. In its simplest form, it involves no more than using standard options within some computerized ANOVA packages to break down the variance into linear and higher order terms. That is, instead of simply estimating the means of all patients at each time point, we first fit a straight line to the means over time, then a quadratic (time^2) term, then a cubic (time^3) term, and so on. If there were repeated observations for a total of k time points, then the data would be fitted with a ($k - 1$) degree polynomial. Thus, in the simplest case where there are only two time points, the best we can do is fit a ($k - 1$) = 1 degree polynomial; i.e. a straight line. As it turns out, a straight line goes rather well through two points.

More complex analysis involves the idea that each person should be fitted separately, since growths are individual (Rogosa *et al.* 1982). Then each parameter of the overall growth curve (the factor, or *beta weight*, multiplying each term) becomes a random variable with its own mean and standard deviation, rather than a point estimate.

To make things more concrete, imagine a series of patients with acute knee injuries enrolled in a physiotherapy programme for treatment. Suppose the therapist aims for biweekly treatments over a total period of three weeks. Table 11.4 shows data for eight such patients.

It is always useful to graph the data prior to analysis, and we have done this in Figure 11.2, which shows the individual data as curves, as well as the means at each time. Examining first the progression of the means, it is evident that they fall on a nearly straight line as a function of time, with a small amount of curvature. This fact suggests that the data could be modelled quite successfully with a linear function, which has only two parameters, the slope and the intercept, and possibly a small quadratic (time^2) term.

We don't usually approach the analysis this way, however. With analysis of variance (ANOVA) or analysis of covariance (ANCOVA), we simply look for differences among means; the data at each time could be interchanged and the results would be the same; the analysis is completely indifferent to the actual functional relationship between time and the dependent variable. In fact, it does

Table 11.4 *Range of motion (in degrees) of knee joints for eight patients enroled in a treatment program at baseline and over five follow-up visits*

Patient	Baseline	Follow-up visit				
		1	2	3	4	5
1	22	23	25	36	42	44
2	30	35	44	51	56	60
3	44	48	50	55	63	66
4	28	32	35	39	42	44
5	40	45	50	57	61	64
6	32	33	35	38	38	37
7	22	27	30	37	42	43
8	40	45	46	55	56	58
Mean	32.25	36.00	39.75	46.00	50.00	52.00

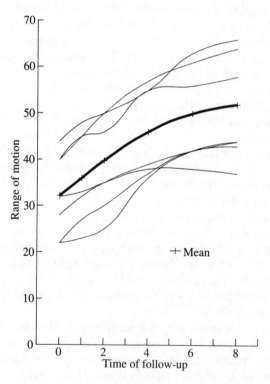

Fig. 11.2. Individual and mean growth curves.

Table 11.5 *Analysis of covariance of range of motion data, with orthogonal decomposition*

Source	Sum of squares	df	Mean square	F	Tail prob
Orthogonal decomposition					
Baseline	2509.26981	1	2509.26981	23.40	0.0029
Patients	643.50519	6	107.25086		
Linear trend	1430.17820	1	1430.17820	52.63	0.0002
Patient $\times$ time^1	190.23034	7	27.17576		
Quadratic trend	65.53945	1	65.53945	39.42	0.0004
Patients $\times$ time^2	11.63924	7	1.66275		
Cubic trend	0.37651	1	0.37651	0.19	0.6759
Patient $\times$ time^3	13.85499	7	1.97928		
Quadratic trend	0.80584	1	0.80584	0.50	0.5041
Patient $\times$ time^4	11.37543	7	1.62506		
Conventional analysis					
Time	1496.90000	4	374.22500	46.14	0.0000
Patient $\times$ time	227.10000	28	8.11071		

not account for the difference in timing of the follow-up visits, since time is treated as simply a categorical variable. What we really want is an analysis which separately tests the degree of linear change, and any other components. We can show this contrast between the two methods by doing the regular ANCOVA and also conducting a second analysis, called an 'orthogonal decomposition', where the linear, quadratic, and higher order polynomials are modelled[2]. The results are shown in Table 11.5.

The orthogonal analysis confirms our observations from the graph. The linear relationship with time is highly significant ($F = 52.63$, $p = 0.0002$); the quadratic term is also highly significant ($F = 39.42$, $p = 0.0004$); and no other terms are significant. Note that the sums of squares are additive, so that the conventional result can be obtained by simply adding up all the trend sums of squares to get

[2] The BMDP package (BioMeDical Programs) does this easily as a specification in the repeated measures ANOVA package (BMDP2V). One need only specify ORTHOGONAL. in the /DESIGN paragraph and specify the particular times using a POINT command to create the output shown.

the overall effect of time; and all the patient × time sums of squares to get the overall patient × time term. This results in a significant overall effect of time; the *F* value is slightly lower, but it is more significant (because the degree of freedom in the numerator is 4 instead of 1).

Why are the results not all that different between the two analyses? In this case, because the individual growth curves are quite different. There is a large patient × time interaction, showing that individual patients are changing at quite different rates. This can be tested manually by taking the ratio of the patient × time interaction (27.17) to the appropriate error term ([11.64 + 13.85 + 11.37]/ 21 = 1.75) resulting in an overall test of the difference in patients in linear trend of (27.17/1.75) = 15.5, which is highly significant. As a result, the gain in statistical power is only marginal.

In general, if all the error variance results from systematic differences in the slopes of individual growth curves (that is, all subjects are changing at different rates), then the overall ANOVA will be more powerful than the trend analysis. Conversely, if all subjects are changing linearly at the same rate, the trend analysis is more powerful.

Modelling individual growth

While the methods outlined above are a more satisfactory strategy for modelling change when multiple observations are available than the use of standard ANOVA methods, they do have a severe restriction. Ordinary analysis software for repeated measures ANOVA, with or without trend analysis, requires a complete data set; all subjects must be measured at the same times and all subjects must have data at each time point. Any missing data will result in the complete loss of the case. This is an obvious constraint when applied to the real world of scattered follow-up visits or repeated assessments. In addition, it appears conceptually unnecessary. We have reconceptualized the problem as one of modelling individual change, using whatever data are available on each subject, then aggregating these data (i.e. the growth parameters) over all subjects. Under this model, it is unnecessarily restrictive to constrain time of assessment to a few standard points.

The solution to the problem is to analyse the data as two regression problems. The first step is to conduct individual regression analyses for each subject, estimating the linear, quadratic, and other higher-order growth parameters. The second step is to then aggregate the parameters across all subjects, essentially treating the growth parameters as random, normally distributed variables. If the goal is to predict individual growth, the parameters are estimated using a second regression equation, where the dependent variable is the growth parameter, and the various predictors (e.g. initial severity, age, fitness) are independent variables. The method is called *hierarchical regression modelling* (Bryk and Raudenbush 1987). Unfortunately, complex software is necessary to conduct this analysis. We are aware of only one standard software package[3] which is capable

---

[3] Again, a new release in BMDP, the BMDP5V program is the program for this analysis.

Table 11.6 *Analysis of individual growth curves using maximum likelihood procedures*

Parameter	Estimate	Asymptotic SE	Z-Score	Two-sided p-value
1 Baseline	70.9203	36.0466	1.967	0.050
2 Linear	4.63821	0.4680	9.911	0.000
3 Quadratic	-0.25805	0.0401	-6.429	0.000

of modelling individual growth parameters as random variable. The method uses maximum likelihood estimation procedures, and as a result does not create the usual ANOVA table; instead, the parameters with their standard errors are estimated directly, similar to a regression analysis. An output from BMDP5V, using the same data set, is shown in Table 11.6:

The *p*-values suggest that the results are similar to those observed previously. This can be confirmed by squaring the Z-scores, which are interpretable as *F* values. Thus, this analysis results in an *F*-test for the baseline measurement of 3.86 (1.967^2) versus 23.40 previously; a linear term of 98.2 (9.911^2) versus the 52.6 observed previously; and an *F*-test for the quadratic term of 41.33 versus 39.42 previously, so we have gained some statistical power using this approach. In general, when the data are complete the results will be similar; however, this method accommodates incomplete data sets.

Summary

This chapter has attempted to resolve some controversies surrounding the measurement of change. There are two distinct purposes for measuring change— examining overall effects of treatments and distinguishing individual differences in treatment response. Focusing on the former, we demonstrated that reliability and sensitivity to change are different but related concepts. We determined the conditions under which the measurement of change will result in increased and decreased statistical power. We also reviewed the literature on the use of change scores to correct for baseline differences and concluded that this purpose can rarely be justified.

As an extension of the methods to measure change, we have considered in detail the use of growth curves in the circumstances where there are more than two observations per subject. The method is conceptually more satisfactory than the classical approach of considering only a beginning and an end point. In addition, growth curve analyses appropriately use all the data available from individual subjects, even when they are measured at different times after the initial assessment.

References

Bryk, A. S. and Raudenbush, S. W. (1987). Application of hierarchical linear models to assessing change. *Psychological Bulletin*, **101**, 147–58.

Burckhardt, C. S., Goodwin, L. D., and Prescott, P. A. (1982). The measurement of change in nursing schools: Statistical considerations. *Nursing Research*, **31**, 53–5.

Conway, M. and Ross, M. (1984). Getting what you want by revising what you had. *Journal of Personality and Social Psychology*, **47**, 738–48.

Cronbach, L. J. and Furby, L. (1970). How should we measure 'change'—or should we? *Psychological Bulletin*, **74**, 68–80.

Francis, D. J., Fletcher, J. M., Stuebing, K. K., Davidson, K. C., and Thompson, N. M. (1991). Analysis of change: Modelling individual growth. *Journal of Consulting and Clinical Psychology*, **59**, 27–37.

Guyatt, G., Walter, S. D., and Norman, G. R. (1987). Measuring change over time: Assessing the usefulness of evaluative instruments. *Journal of Chronic Diseases*, **40**, 171–8.

Linn, P. L. and Slinde, J. A. (1977). Determination of the significance of change between pre- and posttesting periods. *Reviews of Educational Research*, **47**, 121–50.

Linton, S. J. and Melin, L. (1982). The accuracy of remembering chronic pain. *Pain*, **13**, 281–5.

Lord, F. M. (1967). A paradox in the interpretation of group comparisons. *Psychological Bulletin*, **68**, 304–5.

Lord, F. M. and Novick, M. N. (1968). *Statistical theories of mental test development*. Addison-Wesley, Reading, MA.

MacKenzie, C. R., Charlson, M. E., DiGioia, D., and Kelley, K. (1986). Can the Sickness Impact Profile measure change: An example of scale assessment. *Journal of Chronic Diseases*, **39**, 429–38.

McFarland, C. and Ross, M. (1987). The relation between current impressions and memories of dating partners. *Personality and Social Psychology Bulletin*, **13**, 228–38.

McFarland, C., Ross, M., and deCourville, N. (1987). *Women's theories of menstruation and biases in recall of menstrual symptoms*. Unpublished manuscript.

Niemi, G., Katz, R. S., and Newman, D. (1980). Reconstructing past partisanship: The failure of party identification recall questions. *American Journal of Political Science*, **24**, 633–51.

Rogosa, D., Brandt, D., and Zimowski, M. (1982). A growth curve approach to the measurement of change. *Psychological Bulletin*, **92**, 726–48.

Ross, M. (1989). Relation of implicit theories to the construction of personal histories. *Psychological Review*, **96**, 341–57.

Spiro, S. E., Shalev, A., Solomon, Z., and Kotler, M. (1989). Self-reported change versus changed self-report: Contradictory findings of an evaluation of a treatment program for war veterans suffering from post traumatic stress disorder. *Evaluation Review*, **15**, 533–49.

Withey, S. B. (1954). Reliability of recall of income. *Public Opinion Quarterly*, **18**, 157–204.

12

Item Response Theory

Generalizability theory has been the underpinning for most test construction and theory since it was first introduced. One reason for its popularity is that the assumptions that generalizability theory makes about items and test are relatively 'weak' ones, meaning that the theory is appropriate in most situations (Hambleton and Swaminathan 1985). However, there are a number of limitations to generalizability theory (Shea *et al.* 1988). First, as we have pointed out in the chapters on reliability and validity, item and scale statistics apply only to the specific group of subjects who took the test; if the instrument is to be administered to subjects who are different in some way, it is often necessary to re-establish its psychometric properties. Second, it is extremely difficult to compare a person's scores on two or more different tests. The usual approach is to convert the totals to z scores, as we mentioned in Chapter 7. However, this assumes that all of the tests are normally distributed, which is rarely the case (Micceri 1989). The third assumption is that of homoscedasticity; that the error of measurement is the same at the high end of the scale as in the middle or at the low end. This, too, is often an unwarranted assumption, since the errors tend to be smaller near the ends of the range of possible test scores, where 'floor' and 'ceiling' effects come into play. Last, if a person answers 50 per cent of the items in a positive direction, all we can say in traditional test theory is that his or her probability of responding positively to any given item is 50 per cent. The assumption here is that all of the items have equal valences. It is impossible to predict, though, how a person will respond on any given item if the items differ in their propensity to tap the attribute.

Another set of concerns with classic test theory is that it is difficult to separate out the properties of a test from the attributes of the people taking it (Hambleton *et al.* 1991). That is, the scores on an instrument depend on how much of the trait the people in the sample have; while 'how much they have' depends on the norms of the scale. Thus, the instrument's characteristics change as we test different groups, and the groups' characteristics change as we use different tests.

Within the past decade, a different theory of test construction has been proposed which, it is claimed, rectifies these shortcomings. Called *item response theory*, it is based on two 'hard' assumptions: that the data are unidimensional (i.e. the items tap only one trait or ability); and that the probability of answering any item in a positive direction (that is, reflecting more of the trait) is unrelated to the probability of answering any other item positively for people with the

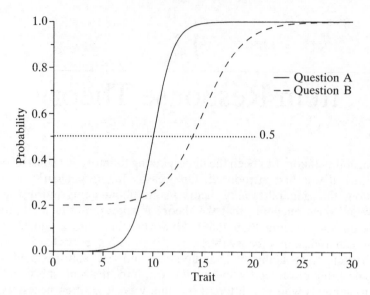

Fig. 12.1. Hypothetical item characteristic curves for two items.

same amount of the trait (a property called 'local independence'). If these assumptions are true (they are testable, although rarely tested), then two postulates follow. First, the performance of a subject on the test can be predicted by a set of factors, which are variously called 'traits', 'abilities', or 'latent traits' (and which are referred to in the theory by the Greek letter, θ, *theta*). The second postulate is that the relationship between a person's performance on any item and the underlying trait can be described by an *item characteristic curve*.

Item characteristic curves

Figure 12.1 depicts hypothetical curves showing the response to two questions, A and B, on a test of some trait. These are called *item characteristic curves* (ICCs). A few important characteristics of the curves are worth noting. They are similar to one another in two ways. First, they are both S shaped (the technical name for the shape is an 'ogive'). While other shapes of the ICC are possible, the ogive is the most widely used one in test construction. Second, they are *monotonic*; the probability of answering in a positive direction consistently increases as the score on the latent trait increases. However, they differ from each other along three dimensions: the steepness of their slopes; their location along the trait continuum; and where they flatten out on the bottom. We shall return to the significance of these differences shortly.

For illustrative purposes, we have drawn a horizontal line where the probability is 0.5; it intersects Question A at value of the trait of 10, and Question B at a value of 14. Strictly speaking, a '50 per cent probability' does *not* mean that a given individual has a 50 per cent chance of responding to the question positively; rather, it means that if we took 100 people with the same amount of the trait, 50 of them will answer one way and 50 the other way. (Models have been developed to handle items with more than two responses, but they are computationally quite difficult, and few computer programs exist to handle these cases.)

What can we tell from these two curves? First, Question A is probably a better discriminator of the trait than Question B. The reason is that the proportion of people responding in the positive direction changes relatively rapidly on Question A as the value of the trait increases. The slope for Question B is flatter, indicating that it does not discriminate as well. For example, as we move from a trait value of 5 to 15, the proportion of people answering positively to Question A increases from 1 per cent to 99 per cent; while for Question B, a comparable 10-point change in the trait is associated with an increase only from 26 per cent to 94 per cent. When the curve has the maximum steepness, it takes the form of a 'step function'; no people below the critical point respond positively, and everyone above it responds in the positive direction. The items would then form a perfect Guttman type of scale. Thus, one way of thinking about item response curves is that they are 'imperfect' Guttman scales, where the probability of responding increases gradually with more of the trait, rather than jumping from a probability of 0 to 100 per cent.

A second observation is that Question B is 'harder' than Question A throughout most of the range of the trait. That is, the average person needs more of the trait in order to respond in the positive direction. This can be seen by the fact that the 50 per cent point is further along the trait continuum for Question B than it is for Question A.

Different models

When item response theory was first developed, a simplifying assumption was made that the ICC ogives were all based on a normal distribution of scores. This assumption has been replaced by three 'models' which are likely more accurate descriptions of the distribution of responses. The simplest is the *one-parameter model*, which is also referred to as the *Rasch model* (Rasch 1960; Wright 1977). According to this model, the only factor affecting the ICCs of the various items in a test is the item difficulty, denoted b_i. That is, it assumes that all of the items have equal discriminating ability (designated as a). This is reflected in that the slopes of all the curves are parallel, but they are placed at various points along the trait continuum, as in Figure 12.2.

Formally, the proportion of people who have θ amount of the trait who answer item i correctly is given as:

$$P_i(\theta) = \frac{\exp\{a(\theta - b_i)\}}{1 + \exp\{a(\theta - b_i)\}}.$$

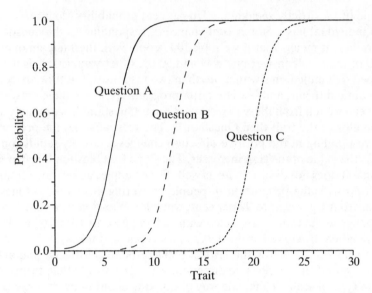

Fig. 12.2. Item characteristic curves for three items with equal discrimination but different levels of difficulty.

Since the form of this equation is called 'logistic', this and the other two models are referred to as *logistic models* or *logistic ogive models*.

The *two-parameter model* holds that the ICCs differ from each other on the basis of both difficulty and discriminating ability; that is, instead of *a* being a constant, there is a different a_i for each item. Now the ICCs differ from each other in two ways; the position along the trait line, and the slope of the curve, as seen in Figure 12.3.

The equation for this takes the form

$$P_i(\theta) = \frac{\exp\{a_i(\theta - b_i)\}}{1 + \exp\{a_i(\theta - b_i)\}}.$$

Both of these models assume that at the lowest level of the trait, the probability of responding positively is zero; that is, the left tail of all of the curves is asymptotic to the *x*-axis. This may be a valid assumption if the test is a personality or attitudinal questionnaire. However, with achievement tests, such as multiple-choice questionnaires, it is likely that people will guess on questions to which they do not know the answer, and get a certain proportion of those items correct by chance. The *three-parameter model* takes this into account, and allows the lower end of the curve to asymptote at some probability level greater than 0. This 'pseudo-guessing parameter' is designated as c_i, and the resulting equation is given as:

$$P_i(\theta) = c_i + \frac{(1 - c_i)\exp\{a_i(\theta - b_i)\}}{1 + \exp\{a_i(\theta - b_i)\}}.$$

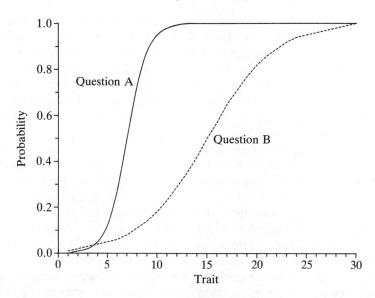

Fig. 12.3. Item characteristic curves for two items differing in both discrimination and difficulty.

An example of a curve where c_i is 0.2 rather than 0.0 is Question B in Figure 12.1.

Deriving the curves

The mechanics of deriving ICCs involve taking a large number of subjects (a minimum of 200 for estimating a one-parameter model, and some authors have recommended using as many as 1000 to estimate the three parameters accurately), for whom we know or can estimate their value of the trait. If we do not have enough information to estimate the trait, then we must make some assumptions about its distribution, and sample people who span the range of the trait. The first step is to calculate the proportion of people at each level of the trait who answer each question in the positive direction. Most computer programs, such as BICAL (Wright *et al.* 1980), which is based on the one-parameter model, or LOGIST (Wingersky 1983), which can estimate the three-parameter one, then determine if the items meet the underlying assumption of unidimensionality. This is most often done by factor analysing the item correlation matrix; unidimensionality would be reflected in a large, dominant first factor, with the remaining factors being relatively weak.

The next step is to decide whether to use a one-, two-, or three-parameter model. While this decision *should* be based on the underlying theory one has about the trait and empirical comparisons of the results, it is more often determined by pragmatic issues: far larger samples are needed to estimate the slope and guessing parameters, and most of the available computer programs are based on the one-parameter Rasch model. With the data for the proportion of people responding positively to each item and the model to be used, the program then can compute the necessary parameters for each item. The specific mathematics of calculating ICCs are beyond the scope of this book, and require a computer if the results are needed in a reasonable time. Those who want to delve deeper into this topic should see Lord (1980).

The latent-trait model differs from the more traditional, random sampling, approach to test construction in a number of ways. With the latter, the items are assumed to be randomly chosen from a universe of possible items, and the person's score is the number of items responded to positively. Each item can thus be seen as, in some sense, equivalent to each other item. The latent-trait model, on the other hand, postulates a known relationship between the response to a specific item and the underlying trait; each item stands alone, having a different difficulty parameter. One trade-off is that for the random sampling approach, it is necessary to start with a large pool of items, but it is not necessary to know much about the items before item selection begins. Far fewer items are needed with the latent-trait approach, but more needs to be known about the item–trait relationship.

Advantages and disadvantages

The major potential advantage of ICC scaling is that it allows *test-free measurement*; that is, people can be compared to one another on the trait even if they took different items! Assume that we have developed a test of physical mobility, using latent-trait theory, and have come up with 30 items which span the range from complete immobility at the low end to unrestricted mobility at the top. These items can be thought of as comprising a Guttman-ordered scale; responding positively to the eighth item, for example, means that the person must have responded positively to the previous seven items. Conversely, if a person answers in the negative direction to item 15, then he or she would not answer positively to any item above number 15. Knowing this, we need not give all of the items to all people, only those items which span the point where the person switches from answering in one direction to answering in the other. That point places the person at a specific point on the mobility continuum. Since an underlying assumption of latent-trait theory is that the test is unidimensional, the point can be directly compared to that of another person, who was given a different subset of the items. In actuality, since the slopes are not vertical as with a Guttman scale, a number of items spanning the critical point must be used.

This form of scaling has received its widest application in achievement testing. Many of the newer tests, such as the revised version of the *Wide Range Achievement Test* (Jastak and Wilkinson 1984), the *Keymath Diagnostic Arithmetic Test*

(Connolly *et al*. 1976), and the *Woodcock Reading Mastery Tests* (Woodcock 1973) have used it, so that people at different levels can be given different items, yet be placed on the same scale at the end. This means that people with less of the trait (e.g. spelling ability) are not frustrated by being given a large number of items which are beyond their ability; nor are people with more of the trait bored by having to spell very easy words like 'cat' or 'run'. In addition to reducing frustration, it also reduces testing time, since candidates do not spend large amounts of time on items which are trivial or beyond their ability. This 'adaptive' or 'tailored' testing is not dependent on item response theory, but is greatly facilitated by it.

Despite these advantages, latent-trait theory has not been widely used in test construction. One primary reason is the relatively large sample size needed to accurately estimate the item parameters. While groups of 1000 may be feasible in developing a test that will be used commercially or used for national certification examinations, it is usually infeasible for research purposes or local applications. A second reason is that, in many situations, the assumptions of the one-parameter Rasch model are difficult to meet. In order to find items with equivalent discrimination parameters and which asymptotically approach 0, a large number of items must be initially tested, obviating one potential advantage of the technique. Third, one of the mathematical assumptions of latent-trait theory is 'local independence'. This holds that, for any given level of the trait, the probabilities $P_i(\theta)$ are independent. This then rules out using questions which are chained (the answer to one is dependent upon the answer to previous items), or where the context created by previous questions affects the response to later items. Last, and perhaps most important, latent-trait theory assumes that the item parameters are the same across samples, especially when these samples are drawn from populations situated at different points along the trait continuum. If the items are tested in a number of different groups, then as Choppin (1976) states, 'eventually every item will show discrepancies; every item can be discarded; no item fits the model exactly' (p. 238).

References

Choppin, B. H. (1976). Recent developments in item banking. In *Advances in psychological and educational measurement* (eds. D. N. M. De Gruitjer and L. J. van der Kamp), pp. 233–45. Wiley, New York.

Connolly, A. J., Nachtman, W., and Pritchett, E. M. (1976). *Keymath Diagnostic Arithmetic Test*. American Guidance Service, Circle Pines, MN.

Hambleton, R. K. and Swaminathan, H. (1985). *Item response theory: Principles and applications*. Kluwer Nijhoff, Boston.

Hambleton, R. K., Swaminathan, H., and Rogers, H. J. (1991). *Fundamentals of item response theory*. Sage, Newbury Park, NJ.

Jastak, S. and Wilkinson, G. S. (1984). *The Wide Range Achievement Test - Revised: Administration manual*. Jastak Associates, Wilmington.

Lord, F. M. (1980). *Application of item response theory to practical testing problems*. Erlbaum, Hillsdale, NJ.

Micceri, T. (1989). The unicorn, the normal curve, and other improbable creatures. *Psychological Bulletin*, **105**, 156–66.

Rasch, G. (1960). *Probabilistic models for some intelligence and attainment tests*. Nielson and Lydiche, Copenhagen.

Shea, J. A., Norcini, J. J., and Webster, G. D. (1988). An application of item response theory to certifying examinations in internal medicine. *Evaluation and the Health Professions*, **11**, 283–305.

Wingersky, M. S. (1983). LOGIST: A program for computing maximum likelihood procedures for logistic test models. In *Applications of item response theory* (ed. R. K. Hambleton), pp. 45–56. Educational Research Institute of British Columbia, Vancouver.

Woodcock, R. W. (1973). *Woodcock Reading Mastery Tests manual*. American Guidance Service, Circle Pines, MN.

Wright, B. D. (1977). Solving measurement problems with the Rasch model. *Journal of Educational Measurement*, **14**, 97–116.

Wright, B. D., Mead, R. J., and Bell, S. R. (1980). *BICAL: Calibrating items with the Rasch model* (Research Memorandum No. 23C). University of Chicago, Department of Education Statistical Laboratory.

13

Methods of administration

Having developed the questionnaire, the next problem is how to administer it. This is an issue which not only affects costs and response rates, but, as we shall see, may influence which questions can be asked and in what format. The three methods commonly used to administer questionnaires are face-to-face interviews, over the telephone, and by mail.

As the cost of microcomputers has come down, scales can now be 'administered' by a computer, with the respondent sitting in front of a terminal. At the present time, this is possible primarily within clinical contexts where the subject is already near the researcher's office, or as part of smaller studies. However, as 'lap top' computers become more powerful, computer presentation will become more prevalent. Each of these methods has its own distinct advantages and disadvantages, which will be discussed in this chapter.

Face-to-face interviews

As the name implies, this method involves a trained interviewer administering the scale or questionnaire on a one-to-one basis, either in an office or, more usually, in the subject's home. The latter setting serves to put the respondents at ease, since they are in familiar surroundings, and may also increase compliance, because the subjects do not have to travel. However, home interviewing involves greater cost to the investigator and the possibility of interruptions, for instance, by telephones or family members.

Advantages

The advantages of face-to-face interviewing begin even before the first question is asked—the interviewer is sure who is responding. This is not the case with telephone or mail administration, since anyone in the household can answer or provide a second opinion for the respondent. In addition, having to respond verbally to another person reduces the number of items omitted by the respondent; it is more difficult to refuse to answer than simply to omit an item on a form (Quine 1985). The interviewer can also determine if the subject is having any difficulty understanding the items, whether due to a poor grasp of the language, limited intelligence, problems in concentration, or boredom. Further, since many immigrants and people with limited education understand the spoken language better than they can read it, and read it better than they can write it, fewer people will be eliminated because of these problems. This method of administration also allows the interviewer to rephrase the question in terms the person may better understand, or to probe for a more complete response. The converse of this, though, is that without sufficient training, the interviewer may distort the meaning of questions.

Another advantage is the flexibility afforded in presenting the items, since questions in an interview can range from 'closed' to 'open'. Closed questions, which require only a number as a response, such as the person's age, number of children, or years of residence, can be read to the subject. If it is necessary for the respondent to choose among three or more alternatives, or to give a Likert-type response, a card with the possible answers could (and most likely *should*) be given to the person so that memory will not be a factor. Open questions can be used to gather additional information, since respondents will generally give longer answers to open-ended questions verbally rather than in writing. This can sometimes be a disadvantage with verbose respondents.

Complicated questionnaires may contain items which are not appropriate for all respondents; men should not be asked how many pregnancies they have had; native-born people when they immigrated; or people who have never been hospitalized when they were last discharged. These questions are avoided with what are called 'skip patterns;' instructions or arrows indicating to the person that he or she should omit a section by skipping to a later portion of the questionnaire. Unless they are very carefully constructed and worded, skip patterns can be confusing to some respondents—and therefore likely to induce errors—if they have to follow these themselves. In contrast, interviewers, because of their training and experience in giving the questionnaire many times, can wend their way through these skip patterns much more readily, and are less likely to make mistakes. Moreover, with the advent of 'lap top' computers, the order of questions and the skip patterns can be programmed to be presented to the interviewer, so that the potential for asking the wrong questions or omitting items is minimized.

Disadvantages

Naturally, there is a cost associated with all of these advantages, in terms of both time and money. Face-to-face interviews are significantly more expensive to administer than any other method. Interviewers must be trained, so that they ask the same questions in the same way, and handle unusual circumstances similarly. In many studies, random interviews are tape-recorded, to ensure that the interviewers' styles have not changed over time; that they have not become lazy or slipshod, or sound bored. This entails further expense, for the tape-recorder itself, and for the supervisor's time to review the session and go over it with the interviewer.

If the interview is relatively short, the interviewer can arrive unannounced.

This, though, takes the chance that the respondent is at home and is willing to be disturbed. The longer the session, the greater the danger that it will be seen as an imposition. For these reasons, especially when an hour or more of the person's time is needed, it is best to announce the visit beforehand, checking the respondent's willingness to participate and arranging a convenient time to come. This requirement imposes the added costs of telephoning, often repeatedly, until an answer is obtained. Further, since many people work during the day, and only evening interviews are convenient, the number of possible interviews that can be done in one day may be limited.

Another potential cost arises if, for instance, English is not the native language for a sizable proportion of the respondents. Not only must the scales and questions be translated into one or more foreign languages (as would be the case, regardless of the format), but bilingual interviewers must be found. This may not be unduly difficult if there are only a few major linguistic cultures (e.g. English and French in Quebec, Spanish in the southwestern United States, Flemish and French in Belgium), but can be more of a problem in cities which attract many immigrants from different countries. There are more languages to take into account and, if immigration has been recent, there may be few people sufficiently bilingual who can be trained as interviewers.

Finally, attributes of the interviewer may affect the responses given. This can be caused by two factors: biases of the interviewer, and his or her social or ethnic characteristics (Weiss 1975). It has been known for a long time that interviewers can subtly communicate what answers they want to hear, often without being aware that they are doing so (e.g. Rice 1929). This is the easier of the two factors to deal with, since it can be overcome with adequate training (Hyman *et al.* 1954). The more difficult problem is that differences between the interviewer and respondent, especially race, also have an effect (Pettigrew 1964; Sattler 1970). During a gubernatorial campaign in the United States, for example, white telephone interviewers found that 43.8 per cent of those polled preferred the black Democratic candidate, while black interviewers found that his level of support was 52.2 per cent, a difference of 8.4 per cent (Finkel *et al.* 1991). The interaction between the perceived race of the interviewer and the background characteristics of the interviewees was even more striking: among Republicans, there was only a 0.5 per cent difference, while Democrats' reported level of support increased 24.2 per cent with Black interviewers. Among those who reported themselves to be 'apolitical', support increased from 16.7 per cent to 63.6 per cent, although the sample size for this group was small. The reasons usually given for this phenomenon include social desirability, deferring to the perceived preferences of the interviewer because of 'interpersonal deference', or 'courtesy to a polite stranger' (Finkel *et al.* 1991). As is obvious from the results of this and other studies (e.g. Meislin 1987), the race of the interviewer can be detected relatively accurately over the telephone, although it is not known whether the subjects respond to the interviewers' accent, speech patterns, inflections, or other verbal cues.

The effect of sex differences is less clear. Female interviewers usually have fewer refusers and higher completion rates than males (Backstrom and Hursh-Cesar 1981; Hornik 1982), which in part may explain why the majority of interviewers are women (Colombotos *et al.* 1968). The responses women elicit may be different from those given to male interviewers, especially when sexual material is being discussed (Hyman *et al.* 1954), but also when the topic of the interview is politics (Hutchinson and Wegge 1991). Furthermore, the differences in response rates seem to occur more with male interviewees than with females.

Age differences between the interviewer and interviewee have not been extensively studied. The general conclusion, though, is that to the degree that it is possible, the two should be as similar as possible, since perceived similarity generally leads to improved communication (Hutchinson and Wegge 1991; Rogers and Bhowmik 1970).

Telephone questionnaires

An alternative to meeting with the subjects in person is to interview them over the telephone. A major advantage is the savings incurred in terms of time and therefore money; in one Canadian study, a home interview cost $16.10, a telephone interview only $7.10 (Siemiatycki 1979). In the past, researchers have avoided this interviewing method because a significant proportion of homes did not have telephones. Moreover, this proportion was not evenly distributed, but was higher in the lower socioeconomic classes. Thus, any survey using the telephone directory as a sampling frame systematically under-represented poorer people. Indeed, the famous prediction in 1936 by the *Literary Digest* that Alf Landon would beat Roosevelt decisively was based on a telephone survey. Unfortunately for the pollsters, more Roosevelt voters than Landon voters did not have phones, leading to a biased sample.

The situation has changed considerably since then, but not always in directions that make it easier for the researcher. On the positive side, most households in North America now have telephones; in 1981, the national average in the U.S. was 93.1 per cent (Marcus and Crane 1986). However, the converse is that a larger number of people have unlisted numbers; close to 20 per cent in 1975 (Glasser and Metzger 1975). Whereas not having a telephone is still more prevalent among the lower social classes, not listing a number is, because of the additional expense, more of a middle-class phenomenon. Surprisingly, the rate of unlisted numbers among the highest income group is about the same as among the lowest (roughly 16 per cent); middle-income people have the highest unlisted rate (Glasser and Metzger 1975).

Random digit dialling

A technique has been developed to get around this problem of unlisted numbers, called *random digit dialling*. A computer-driven device dials telephone numbers at random, using either all seven digits of the number, or the last four once the three-digit exchange has been chosen by the researcher. This latter refinement was added because some exchanges consist primarily of businesses, whereas others are located in mainly residential neighbourhoods; in some areas, 80 per cent of numbers are not assigned to households (Glasser and Metzger 1972). Pre-selecting the exchange has resulted in an increase in the proportion of households reached with this technique, although it is may still not exceed 50 per cent (Waksberg 1978). One disadvantage of sampling by telephone number rather than by address or name is that homes with more than one telephone have multiple chances of being selected, a bias favouring more affluent households. Another disadvantage is that, since the selected numbers tend to be physically near one another, households tend to be more homogeneous than with a purely random sample. To overcome this 'design effect' due to cluster randomization, larger sample sizes are needed (Waksberg 1978).

Advantages

Many of the advantages of face-to-face interviewing also pertain to telephone surveys. These include (1) a reduction in the number of omitted items; (2) skip patterns are followed by the trained interviewer rather than the respondent; (3) open-ended questions can be asked; (4) a broad, representative sample can be obtained; (5) the interviewer can be prompted by a computer (a technique often referred to as CATI, or Computer Assisted Telephone Interviewing); and (6) the interviewer can determine if the person is having problems understanding the language in general or a specific question in particular.

Another advantage of telephone interviewing is that, even when the person is not willing to participate, he or she may give some basic demographic information, such as age, marital status, or education. This allows the researcher to determine if there is any systematic bias among those who decline to participate in the study.

Moreover, there are at least three areas in which the telephone may be superior to face-to-face interviews. First, any bias which may be caused by the appearance of the interviewer, due to factors such as skin colour or physical deformity, is eliminated. However, one interviewer characteristic which cannot be masked by a telephone is gender. There is some evidence that male interviewers elicit more feminist responses from women and more conservative answers from men than do female interviewers; and more optimistic reports from both sexes regarding the economic outlook (Groves and Fultz 1985). These authors also report higher refusal rates for male interviewers, which is consistent with other studies.

A second advantage is that nationwide surveys can be conducted out of one office, which lowers administrative costs and facilitates supervision of the interviewers to ensure uniformity of style. Last, there is some evidence that people may report more health-related events in a telephone interview than in a face-to-face one (Thornberry 1987), although it is not clear that the higher figure is necessarily more accurate.

Disadvantages

A potential problem with telephone interviewing is that another person in the household may be prompting the respondent. However, this risk is fairly small, since the person on the phone would have to repeat each question aloud. A more difficult issue is that there is no assurance who the person is at the other end of the line. If the sampling scheme calls for interviewing the husband, for instance, the masculine voice can be that of the chosen respondent's son or father. This may be a problem if the designated person is an immigrant unsure of his or her grasp of the language and asks a more fluent member of the household to substitute.

Another difficulty with telephone interviews, as with face-to-face ones, is that unless a specific respondent is chosen beforehand, the sample may be biased by *when* the call is made. During the day, there is a higher probability that house-wives, shift workers, the ill, or the unemployed will be reached. Evening calls may similarly bias the sample by excluding shift workers. Traugott (1987) found that people reached during the day did not differ significantly from those who could be contacted only in the evening with respect to age, race, or sex; but that the latter group were more likely to be college graduates, since they tended to be employed and not work shifts.

A major problem with telephone interviewing, as opposed to face-to-face interviewing, is the difficulty with questions which require the person to choose among various options. With the interviewer present, he or she can hand the respondent a card listing the response alternatives; an option not available over the telephone. A few suggestions have been offered to overcome this problem. The easiest to implement is to have to respondent write the alternatives on a piece of paper, and then to refer to them when answering. This is feasible when one response set is used with a number of items, such as a Likert scale which will be referred to in responding to a set of questions. However, if each item requires a different list, the method can become quite tedious and demanding, and the respondent may either hang up or not write the alternatives down, relying on his or her (fallible) memory. In the latter situation, a 'primacy effect' is likely to occur, with subjects tending to endorse categories that are read toward the beginning rather than toward the end of the list (Locander and Burton 1976; Monsees and Massey 1979).

A second method is to divide the question into parts, with each section prob-ing for a more refined answer. For example, the person can be asked if he or she agrees or disagrees with the statement. Then the next question would tap the strength of the endorsement: mild or strong. It also helps if the response format is given to the person as an introduction to the question; for example, 'In the fol-lowing question, there will be four possible answers: strongly agree, mildly agree, mildly disagree, and strongly disagree. The question is . . .'.

A third method involves a pre-interview mailing to the subjects. This can con-sist of the entire questionnaire itself, or a card with the response alternatives.

With the former, the interviewer then reads each question, with the respondent following in his or her version. The telephone call allows for probing and recording answers to open-ended questions. If a card with the alternatives is mailed, it is often combined with features like emergency telephone numbers or other items which encourage the person to keep it near the telephone, readily available when the call comes (Aneshensel *et al.* 1982).

These various techniques make it more feasible to ask complicated questions over the telephone. However, the major consideration with this form of interviewing remains to reduce complexity as much as possible. If detailed explanations are necessary, as may be the case if the person's attitudes toward public policy issues are being evaluated, face-to-face or mailed questionnaires may be preferable.

Whatever technique is used, it is highly likely that repeated calls may be necessary to reach a desired household; people may be working, out for the evening, in hospital, or on vacation. It has been recommended that three to six attempts may be required; after this, the law of diminishing returns begins to play an increasingly large role. Moreover, the call should not be made at times such that the respondents feel it would be an intrusion: on holidays, Sundays, or during major sports events.

Mailed questionnaires

Advantages

Mailing questionnaires to respondents is by far the cheapest method of the three; in Siemiatycki's study (1979), the average cost was $6.08, as opposed to $7.10 for telephone interviewing and $16.10 for home interviewing. In the past, the major drawback has been a relatively low response rate, jeopardizing the generalizability of the results. Over the years, various techniques have been developed which have resulted in higher rates of return. Dillman (1978), one of the most ardent spokesmen for this interviewing method, has combined many of them into what he calls the *Total Design Method*. He believes that response rates of over 75 per cent are possible with a general mailing to a heterogeneous population, and of 90 per cent to a targeted group, such as family practitioners.

As with telephone interviews, mailed questionnaires can be coordinated from one central office, even for national or international studies. In contrast, personal interviews usually require an office in each major city, greatly increasing the expense. Further, since there is no interviewer present, either in person or at the other end of a telephone line, social desirability bias tends to be minimized.

Disadvantages

However, there are a number of drawbacks with this method of administration. First, if a subject does not return the questionnaire, it is almost impossible to get any demographic information, obviating the possibility of comparing responders with non-responders. Second, subjects may omit some of the items; it is quite common to find statements in articles to the effect that 5 to 10 per cent of the returned questionnaires were unusable due to omitted, illegible, or invalid responses (e.g. Nelson *et al.* 1986). Third, while great care may have been taken by the investigator with regard to the sequence of the items, there is no assurance that the subjects read them in order. Some people may skip to the end first, or delay answering some questions because they have difficulty interpreting them.

A fourth difficulty is that, to ensure a high response rate (over 80 per cent), it is often necessary to send out two or three mailings to some subjects. If the identity of the respondent is known, then this necessitates some form of bookkeeping system, to record who has returned the questionnaire and who should be sent a reminder. If anonymity is desired, then reminders and additional copies must be sent to all subjects, increasing the cost of the study. Fifth, there may be a delay of up to three months until all the questionnaires that will be returned have been received. Last, there is always the possibility that some or all of the questionnaires may be delayed by a postal strike.

Increasing the return rate

Many techniques have been proposed to increase the rate of return of mailed questionnaires, although not all have proven to be effective. These have included:

1. *A covering letter.* Perhaps the most important part of a mailed questionnaire is the letter accompanying it. It will determine if the form will be looked at or thrown away, and the attitude with which the respondent will complete it. A detailed description of letters and the contents is given by Dillman (1978), who stresses their importance. The letter should begin with a statement which emphasizes two points: why the study is important; and why that person's responses are necessary to make the results interpretable, in that order. Common mistakes are to indicate in the opening paragraph that a questionnaire (a word he says is to be avoided) is enclosed; that it is part of a survey (another 'forbidden' word); identifying who the researcher is before stating why the research is being done; or under whose auspices (again, best left for later in the letter). Other points that should be included in the letter are a promise of confidentiality, a description of how the results will be used, and a mention of any incentive. The letter should be signed by hand, with the name block under the signature indicating the person's title and affiliation. Since subjects are more likely to respond if the research is being carried out by a university or some other respected organization, its letterhead should be used whenever it is appropriate. The letter itself should fit onto one page; coloured paper may look more impressive, but does not appear to influence the response rate.

2. *Advance warning that the questionnaire will be coming.* A letter is seen as less

of an intrusion than a form which has to be completed, especially one that arrives unannounced. The introductory letter thus prepares the respondent for the questionnaire, and helps differentiate it from junk mail. Unfortunately for the researcher, many 'give away' offers now use the same technique; an official-looking letter announcing the imminent arrival of a packet of chances to win millions of dollars. This makes the wording of the covering letter even more critical, in order to overcome the scepticism that often greets such unsolicited arrivals.

3. *Giving a token of appreciation in advance*. Most often, this is a sum of money. Up to about $3.00, the actual amount does not appear to affect the response rate, although giving something is far better than nothing (Fox *et al.* 1988; Yu and Cooper 1983). Over $3.00, there is a very strong positive relationship between the size of the gift and the proportion of forms which are returned, although the number of studies on which this conclusion is based is quite small. It is not worth the effort to *promise* an incentive; if the reward is not included with the questionnaire, the response rate will be about the same as if no inducement were offered (Church 1993). Other incentives which have been used successfully have included lottery tickets, pens or pencils (a favourite among census bureaus), tie clips, unused stamps, diaries, donations to charity, key rings, golf balls, and letter openers. Although offering to send the respondent the results of the completed study is often used as a reward, especially in academia, it does not appear to have any effect on response rate (Yu and Cooper 1983). The objective of enclosing an incentive is to acknowledge that completing the questionnaire costs the person time and effort, which is appreciated and partially compensated by the gift. It often helps to spell this out explicitly in a covering letter, indicating that the reward can be only a token of thanks.

4. *Anonymity*. The literature on the effect of anonymity on response rate is contradictory. If the person is identifiable on questionnaires which ask for confidential information, such as income, sexual practices, or illegal acts, then the response rate is definitely jeopardized. However, promises of confidentiality for non-sensitive material does not appear to materially increase compliance; although it is probably safest to ensure anonymity. If it is necessary to identify the respondent, in order to link the responses to other information or to determine who should receive follow-up reminders, then the purpose of the identification should be stated, along with guarantees that the person's name will be thrown away when it is no longer needed, and kept under lock and key in the meantime; and that in the final report, no subject will be identifiable.

5. *Personalization*. Envelopes addressed to 'Occupant' are often regarded as junk mail, and are either discarded unopened, or read in a cursory manner; the same may be true of the salutation on the letter itself. However, some people see a personalized greeting using their name as an invasion of privacy and a threat to anonymity. This problem can be handled in a number of ways. First, the letter can be addressed to a group, such as 'Dear Colleague', 'Resident of . . . Neighbourhood', or 'Member of . . . '; the personalization is given with a handwritten

signature. (Again, with the wide use by politicians and advertisers of machines which produce signatures which resemble handwriting, this may become less effective with time.) Another method to balance anonymity and personalization is to have the covering letter personalized, and to stress the fact that the questionnaire itself has no identifying information on it.

Other aspects of personalization include typed addresses rather than labels, stamps rather than metered envelopes, and regular envelopes rather than business reply ones. The former alternatives are usually associated with junk mail, and the latter with important letters. Based on their meta-analysis of 34 published and unpublished studies, Armstrong and Lusk (1987) found that stamped, first-class mail had a return rate on average of 9.2 per cent higher than when business replies were used. Interestingly, using a number of small-denomination stamps on the envelope yielded slightly better results (by 3.5 per cent) than using one stamp with the correct postage.

6. *Enclosing a stamped, self-addressed envelope.* Asking the respondents to complete the questionnaire is an imposition on their time; asking them to also find and address a return envelope and pay for the postage is a further imposition, guaranteed to lead to a high rate of non-compliance. In what appears to be the only empirical study of this, Ferriss (1951) obtained a response rate of 90.1 per cent with an enclosed stamped return envelope; this dropped to 25.8 per cent when the envelope was omitted. Surprisingly, the "active ingredient" seems to be the envelope itself, rather than the stamp. Armstrong and Lusk (1987), after reviewing six articles comparing stamped versus unstamped return envelopes, found a difference of only 3 per cent in favour of using stamps.

7. *Length of the questionnaire.* It seems logical that shorter questionnaires should lead to higher rates of return than longer ones. However, the research shows that length is a relatively weak factor in comparison to others (Yu and Cooper 1983). When the questionnaire is long (over roughly 100 items or 10 pages), each additional page reduces the response rate by about 0.4 per cent. Up to that point, the content of the questionnaire is a far more potent factor affecting whether or not the person will complete it (Goyder 1982; Heberlein and Baumgartner 1978). In fact, there is some evidence that lengthening the questionnaire by adding interesting questions may actually increase compliance and lead to more valid answers (Dillman 1978; Burchell and Marsh 1992). Thus, it seems that once a person has been persuaded to fill out the form, its length is of secondary importance.

8. *Pre-coding the questions.* Although this does not appear to appreciably increase compliance, pre-coding does serve a number of useful purposes. First, open-ended questions must at some point be coded for analysis; in other words, coding must take place at one time or another. Second, subjects are more likely to check a box rather than write out a long explanation. Last, handwritten responses may be illegible or ambiguous. On the other hand, subjects may feel that they want to explain their answers, or indicate why none of the alternatives apply (a sign of a poorly designed question). The questionnaire can make pro-

visions for this, having optional sections after each section or at the end for the respondent to add comments.

9. *Follow-ups.* As important as the letter introducing the study is the follow-up to maximize returns. Dillman (1978) outlines a four-step process:

- Seven to ten days after the first mailing, a postcard should be sent, thanking those who have returned the questionnaire, and reminding the others of the study's importance. The card should also indicate to those who have mislaid the original where they can get another copy of the questionnaire.

- Two to three weeks later, a second letter is sent, again emphasizing why that person's responses are necessary for this important study. Also included are another questionnaire and return envelope. This can lead to a problem, though, if it is sent to all subjects, irrespective of whether or not they sent in the first form; very compliant or forgetful subjects may complete two of them.

- The third step, which is not possible in all countries, is to send yet another letter, questionnaire, and envelope via registered or special delivery mail. The former alternative is less expensive, but some people may resent having to make a special trip to the post office for something of no direct importance to them.

- The last step, often omitted because of the expense, is to call those who have not responded to the previous three reminders. This may be impractical for studies which span the entire country, but may be feasible for more local ones.

Some researchers have maintained that while the individual effect of each of these procedures may be slight (with the exception of the initial letter, return envelope, and follow-up, where major effects are seen), their cumulative effect is powerful.

The necessity of persistence

Even when all the techniques are used to maximize the return rate of a mailed questionnaire or to talk to the designated respondent on the telephone, the initial response rate is usually too low to permit accurate conclusions to be drawn. Consequently, most surveys call for follow-up mailings or calls in order to contact most of the subjects. The experience of one typical telephone survey is presented in Figure 13.1, based on data from Traugott (1987). After three follow-up calls, about two-thirds of the respondents were contacted; one particularly elusive person required a total of 30 calls before he was reached.

The necessity of persistence in follow-up has been demonstrated in a number of studies which have shown that people who are easier to contact are different in some important ways from those who are more difficult to find or who require more reminders before they return a questionnaire. Traugott (1987) found that

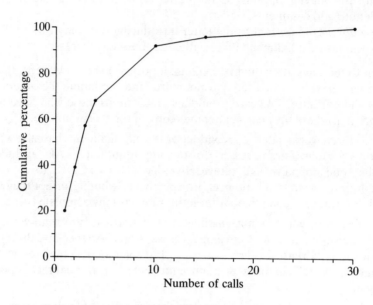

Fig. 13.1. Cumulative contact rate as a function of the number of telephone calls.

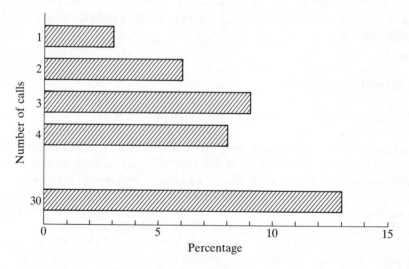

Fig. 13.2. Reagan's lead over Mondale in 1984, as a function of the number of calls required to reach the respondent.

during the 1984 Presidential campaign, Democrats were more accessible than Republicans. As Figure 13.2 shows, people who were found after one telephone call favoured Reagan by 3 per cent; the lead increased to nine points when the sample included people who were reached after three calls; and the total sample gave Reagan a 13-point advantage. He concluded that 'through persistence, the sample became younger and more male' (p. 53). Rao (1983) and Converse and Traugott (1986) summarize a number of different characteristics which are different between early and late responders. The conclusion is that any survey is suspect which bases its results solely on responders to initial mailings or first telephone calls.

Computer-assisted administration

Microcomputers are now ubiquitous, found in most offices and many homes. There are now computers small enough to be placed on one's lap, which rival the power of the original mainframes. Within the past few years, it has become feasible to present even the longest questionnaires on these portable machines. Whereas just a few years ago, computer-administered questionnaires had to be given in the researcher's office, the situation has since changed, and computer-assisted interviewing (CAI) is now fairly commonplace.

Advantages

There are at least four major advantages to computerized administration. First, it can free the interviewer to do other things, or to administer the scale to a number of people simultaneously. Second, every time data are transferred from one medium to another, there is the potential for transcription and entry errors. When the subject is interviewed in person, there are many steps where these errors can creep in: the subject means to say one answer but gives another; the interviewer mishears the response; means to write one thing but puts down something else; errs in transcribing a check mark in one box to a number; or finally keys the wrong number into the computer. Having the person enter his or her responses directly into the machine eliminates all sources of error but one—unknowingly hitting the wrong key. With so many steps eliminated, there is also a commensurate saving of time and money to the researcher.

A third advantage is that neither the subject nor the interviewer can inadvertently omit items or questions. As we have already discussed, a related advantage is that the skip patterns can be automated, eliminating another source of error.

Last, people may be more honest in reporting unacceptable or undesirable behaviours to an impersonal machine than to a human. A number of studies have shown that people admit to more drinking when seated in front of a computer console than an interviewer (e.g. Lucas *et al.* 1977; Skinner and Allen 1983).

Disadvantages

One potential disadvantage of computerizing scales stems from the direct transfer of existing instruments to a computerized format. In most cases, it has not been established whether or not the translation has adversely affected their reliability and validity. Paper-and-pencil questionnaires allow subjects to see how many items there are and to pace themselves accordingly; to skip around, rather than answering the questions in sequence; and to go back easily to earlier questions, in order to change them or to check for their own consistency. While scale developers may deplore these deviations from the way the instrument was intended to be taken, the results of the original reliability and validity studies were conducted with these factors possibly playing a role. Modifying these factors *may* affect the psychometric properties of the scale; the data are not available yet (Green 1984; Moreland 1987).

A second, again potential, disadvantage is the belief, especially among health care workers, that some subjects or patients may be apprehensive about computers. These machines still retain the mystique of 'giant brains' which can, nevertheless, be brought to their knees by the press of a wrong key. However, their apprehension about subjects' reactions to these machines are probably not well founded. Most studies have found that far more people are comfortable in front of a terminal or microcomputer than are uncomfortable. Indeed, in many studies, a majority of responders preferred the machine to a human (see Stein 1987 for a review of this.) A related problem is that attitudes toward computerized interviewing may be sex-related; men tend to be more comfortable 'talking' to machines about sensitive material than to a human interviewer, while the reverse is true for women (e.g. Skinner and Allen 1983). At present, there is insufficient information to indicate whether this is due to the greater use of computers by men, or whether this attitude transcends familiarity with the machines. In either case, though, the sex difference tends to be small.

Implementation

In implementing a computerized scale or questionnaire, some considerations should be kept in mind. First, there should be an ability for the subject to interrupt the testing, and return later to the place where he or she stopped, without either losing the original data or having to go through questions already answered. This is particularly true for long scales, when it is one of many scales, or when the person may become tired or distracted easily. Second, there must be a provision for the subjects to modify their answers, both to the item they are completing at the time, and to previous ones. Respondents should be able to review their earlier answers, modify them if desired, and return to the same place in the instrument. Last, there must be a way for the subject to indicate that he or she cannot or does not want to answer a question. This option is often missing on paper-and-pencil questionnaires, since the person can simply leave the offending item out. If the subject cannot proceed to the next question without entering some response into the machine, the option must be explicit. When he was in the university town of Madison, Wisconsin, one of the pioneers in computerized interviewing, Warner Slack (cited in Fishman 1981), used the phrase 'None of your damn business' as the option the person could use to avoid a question. This was changed to 'Skip that one' when Slack moved to Boston, emphasizing the importance of cultural factors.

In summary, there is no one method of administration that is ideal in all circumstances. Factors such as cost, completion rate, and the type of question asked must all be taken into account. The final decision will, to some degree, be a compromise, in that the disadvantages of the technique that is chosen are outweighed by the positive elements.

References

Aneshensel, C. S., Frerichs, R. R., Clark, V. A., and Yokopenic, P. A. (1982). Measuring depression in the community: A comparison of telephone and personal interviews. *Public Opinion Quarterly*, **46**, 110–21.

Armstrong, J. S. and Lusk, E. J. (1987). Return postage in mail surveys: A meta-analysis. *Public Opinion Quarterly*, **51**, 233–48.

Backstrom, C. H. and Hursh-Cesar, G. (1981). *Survey research* (2nd edn.). Wiley, New York.

Burchell, B. and Marsh, C. (1992). The effect of questionnaire length on survey response. *Quality and Quantity*, **26**, 233–44.

Church, A. H. (1993). Estimating the effect of incentives on mail survey response rates: A meta-analysis. *Public Opinion Quarterly*, **57**, 62–79.

Colombotos, J., Elinson, J., and Loewenstein, R. (1968). Effect of interviewers' sex on interview responses. *Public Health Reports*, **83**, 685–90.

Converse, P. E. and Traugott, M. W. (1986). Assessing the accuracy of polls and surveys. *Science*, **234**, 1094–98.

Dillman, D. A. (1978). *Mail and telephone surveys: The total design method*. Wiley, New York.

Ferriss, A. L. (1951). A note on stimulating response to questionnaires. *American Sociological Review*, **16**, 247–9.

Finkel, S. E., Guterbock, T. M., and Borg, M. J. (1991). Race-of-interviewer effects in a preelection poll: Virginia 1989. *Public Opinion Quarterly*, **55**, 313–30.

Fishman, K. D. (1981). *The computer establishment*. Harper and Row, New York.

Fox, R. J., Crask, M. R., and Kim, J. (1988). Mail survey response rate: A meta-analysis of selected techniques for inducing response. *Public Opinion Quarterly*, **52**, 467–91.

Glasser, G. J. and Metzger, G. D. (1972). Random digit dialling as a method of telephone sampling. *Journal of Marketing Research*, **9**, 59–64.

Glasser, G. J. and Metzger, G. D. (1975). National estimates of nonlisted telephone households and their characteristics. *Journal of Marketing Research*, **12**, 359–61.

Goyder, J. C. (1982). Further evidence on factors affecting response rate to mailed questionnaires. *American Sociological Review*, **47**, 550–3.

Green, B. F. (1984). *Computer-based ability testing*. American Psychological Association, Washington DC.

Groves, R. M. and Fultz, N. H. (1985). Gender effects among telephone interviewers in a survey of economic attitudes. *Sociological Methods and Research*, **14**, 31–52.

Heberlein, T. A. and Baumgartner, R. (1978). Factors affecting response rate to mailed questionnaires: A quantitative analysis of the published literature. *American Sociological Review*, **43**, 447–62.

Hornik, J. (1982). Impact of pre-call request form and gender interaction on response to a mail survey. *Journal of Marketing Research*, **19**, 144–51.

Hutchinson, K. L. and Wegge, D. G. (1991). The effects of interviewer gender upon response in telephone survey research. *Journal of Social Behavior and Personality*, **6**, 573–84.

Hyman, H. H., Cobb, W. J., Feldman, J. J., Hart, C. W., and Stember, C. H. (1954). *Interviewing in social research*. University of Chicago Press, Chicago.

Locander, W. B. and Burton, J. P. (1976). The effect of question form on gathering income data by telephone. *Journal of Marketing Research*, **13**, 189–92.

Lucas, R. W., Mullin, P. J., Luna, C. B. X., and McInroy, D. C. (1977). Psychiatrists and a computer as interrogators of patients with alcohol-related illness: A comparison. *British Journal of Psychiatry*, **131**, 160–67.

Marcus, A. C. and Crane, L. A. (1986). Telephone surveys in public health research. *Medical Care*, **24**, 97–112.

Meislin, R. (1987). Racial divisions seen in poll on Howard Beach attack. *New York Times*, January 8.

Monsees, M. L. and Massey, J. T. (1979). Adapting a procedure for collecting demographic data in a personal interview to a telephone interview. *Proceedings of the American Statistical Association, Social Statistics Section*, 130–5.

Moreland, K. L. (1987). Computerized psychological assessment: What's available. In *Computerized psychological assessment* (ed. J. N. Butcher), pp. 26–49. Basic Books, New York.

Nelson, N., Rosenthal, R., and Rosnow, R. L. (1986). Interpretation of significance levels and effect sizes by psychological researchers. *American Psychologist*, **41**, 1299–301.

Pettigrew, T. F. (1964). *A profile of the Negro American*. Van Nostrand, Princeton, NJ.

Quine, S. (1985). 'Does the mode matter?': A comparison of three modes of questionnaire completion. *Community Health Studies*, **9**, 151–6.

Rao, P. S. R. S. (1983). Callbacks, follow-ups, and repeated telephone calls. In *Incomplete data in sample surveys. Vol. 2: Theory and bibliographies* (eds. W. G. Madow, I. Olkin, and D. B. Rubin), pp. 33–44. Academic Press, New York.

Rice, S. A. (1929). Contagious bias in the interview. *American Journal of Sociology*, **35**, 420–3.

Rogers, E. M. and Bhowmik, D. K. (1970). Homophily–heterophily: Relational concepts for communication research. *Public Opinion Quarterly*, **34**, 523–38.

Sattler, J. (1970). Racial 'experimenter effects' in experimentation, interviewing and psychotherapy. *Psychological Bulletin*, **73**, 137–60.

Siemiatycki, J. (1979). A comparison of mail, telephone, and home interview strategies for household health surveys. *American Journal of Public Health*, **69**, 238–45.

Skinner, H. A. and Allen, B. A. (1983). Does the computer make a difference? Computerized versus face-to-face versus self-report assessment of alcohol, drug, and tobacco use. *Journal of Consulting and Clinical Psychology*, **51**, 267–75.

Stein, S. J. (1987) Computer-assisted diagnosis for children and adolescents. In *Computerized psychological assessment* (ed. J. N. Butcher), pp. 145–58. Basic Books, New York.

Thornberry, O. T. (1987). An experimental comparison of telephone and personal health interview surveys. *Vital and Health Statistics*. Series 2, No. 106. DHHS Pub. No. (PHS) 87-1380.

Traugott, M. W. (1987). The importance of persistence in respondent selection for preelection surveys. *Public Opinion Quarterly*, **51**, 48–57.

Waksberg, J. (1978). Sampling methods for random digit dialling. *Journal of the American Statistical Association*, **73**, 40–6.

Weiss, C. H. (1975). Interviewing in evaluation research. In *Handbook of evaluation research*, Vol. 1 (eds. E. L. Struening and M. Guttentag), pp. 355–95. Sage Publications, Beverly Hills.

Yu, J. and Cooper, H. (1983). A quantitative review of research design effects on response rates to questionnaires. *Journal of Marketing Research*, **20**, 36–44.

14

Ethical Considerations

For the most part, ethical discussions concerning the development and administration of tests have centred around assessments conducted within clinical, educational, or employment settings, and where the results would directly affect the person being evaluated. These situations would include, for example, intelligence, achievement, and aptitude testing in schools; personality and neurocognitive evaluations of patients; and ability testing of job applicants.

Initially, the major focus of the professional organizations was on establishing standards for the tests themselves. In 1895, the American Psychological Association (APA) began looking at the feasibility of standardizing "mental" and physical tests (Novick 1981). The first formal set of guidelines appeared in 1954—the *Technical Recommendations for Psychological Tests and Diagnostic Techniques*, published by the APA—and these were followed a year later by the *Technical Recommendations for Achievement Tests*, prepared by the American Educational Research Association (AERA) and the National Council on Measurement in Education (NCME). These two sets of Recommendations set standards for the assessment and reporting of the psychometric properties of tests, and for the first time set forth the requirements for reliability and validity testing. Later revisions modernized the definitions of reliability and validity, and put greater emphasis on the qualifications of the test user.

Tests which are used only for research purposes, however, are usually considered to be exempt from these standards. This does not mean that there are no ethical problems in devising and using instruments for primarily research questions. Consider the following situations:

Example A. While filling out a questionnaire enquiring about various mood states, one respondent writes in the margin of the answer sheet that she is feeling very despondent, and has recently been thinking of taking her own life. Another subject, while not as explicit about his suicidal thoughts, scores in a range indicative of severe emotional turmoil.

Example B. You are developing a test of marital relationships, and have assured the respondents that their answers will remain confidential, especially since some of the items tap issues of infidelity. One year later, the spouse of one of the respondents files for a divorce, and subpoenas the questionnaire to be used as evidence in court.

Example C. In order to validate a self-report measure of medical utilization, you need to examine the charts of subjects to see how much use they make of various hospital services. In order to ensure that the results are not biased by those who refused to participate in the study, you want to pull their charts to obtain some basic demographic information about them, and to determine their use of medical services.

Example D. Your aim is to develop a measure of self-esteem. One validity study would involve testing two groups of students before and after they make an oral presentation. Subjects in one group are told that they did very well, and those in the other group that they had done very badly and had made fools of themselves, irrespective of how they actually had performed. The students were enrolled in an Introductory Psychology class, and had to participate in three studies as part of the course requirements.

Example E. In order to develop a test of abstract reasoning ability, it is necessary to administer it to people ranging in age from five to 75, and to psychiatric patients who may exhibit problems in this area, such as schizophrenics and those with brain injuries.

These situations illustrate a number of ethical considerations which may be encountered, such as the use of deception, confidentiality, free and informed consent, and the proper balance between the researcher's need for data and the individual's right to privacy. In this section, we will discuss these and other issues, and see how they affect scale development. As with many aspects of ethics, there are few right or wrong answers. Rather, there are general considerations which must be weighed and balanced against each other, and the "correct" approach may vary from one situation and institution to another.

The primary consideration in all discussions of ethics is *respect for the individual's autonomy.* This means that we treat people in such a way that they can decide for themselves whether or not to participate in a study. At first glance, this principle may seem so self-evident that one wonders why it is even mentioned; it appears as if it should be understood and accepted by everyone, both researchers and subjects. However, the implementation of the principle of autonomy can lead to some thorny issues.

To begin with, people cannot exercise autonomy unless they know what it is that they are agreeing to. This means that there must be *informed consent*; that is, the subjects must be told (a) that they are participating in a research study, (b) what the study is about, and (c) what they are being called upon to do. In studies done for the purpose of scale development, these requirements are most often easy to meet and present no difficulties.

Example D, though, involves deception, in that the subjects are not told that the feedback about their performance is fallacious. Indeed, it could be argued that the study would be impossible if the students were told its true nature. Wilson and Donnerstein (1976) give examples of at least eight types of studies in which they feel deception was a necessary and integral part. Some professional organizations—mainly medical ones, which have little experience with psychosocial research methods—have a blanket prohibition against all studies which involve deception; and some people have argued that it is always possible to substitute observational procedures which do not involve deception for experiments which do (e.g., Shipley 1977). Others, such as the APA and the Medical Research Council of Canada (MRC), discourage its use, but recognize that there are some situations where it is required. If no alternative research strategy is possible, then the APA and MRC state that (a) the subjects must be told of the deception after their participation, and (b) the researcher must be able to cope with any possible psychological sequelae which may result from the deception (American Psychological Association 1992; Medical Research Council of Canada 1987).

A different problem with free and informed consent is raised in Example E. How "informed" can the consent be from minors or those whose cognitive processes are compromised because of some innate or acquired disorder? Some ethicists have argued that those who are unable to fully comprehend the nature of the study and to refuse to participate should never be used in research studies unless they benefit directly from their participation; even parents should not be able to give surrogate consent for their children. Adoption of this extreme view, though, would result in "research orphans"; groups on whom no research can be done, even if it may result in potential benefit to other members of that group.

Although few people adhere to such an extreme position, it is widely recognized that special precautions must be taken with these vulnerable groups. For those who are legally minors (the age of majority varies between 16 and 18, depending on the jurisdiction), the consent of at least one parent is mandatory. Increasingly over the years, there has been legal recognition of a grey zone between the age of majority and some vaguely defined point where the child is capable of understanding that he or she is part of a study. Within this age frame, the child's *assent* is required in addition to the parent's consent. This means that the child must not object to being in the study, although actively saying "I agree" is not necessary. If he or she does object, this overrides the consent of the parent. Unfortunately for the investigator, the lower age of this zone is rarely explicitly stated, in recognition of the fact that children mature at different rates; it is left to the judgement of the researcher to determine if the child is cognitively capable of understanding.

A rational guideline for what can be done with children is provided by the *Guidelines* of the MRC (1987). It states that:

...society and parents should not expose children to greater risks, for the sake of pure medical research, than the children take in their everyday lives... Parents may consent to inspection of their children's medical records for research... (p. 29).

Psychiatric patients pose a different set of problems. Having a diagnosed disorder such as schizophrenia does not necessarily mean that the person is incompetent and unable to give consent (or to deny it). Some institutions have taken the position that some mental health worker who does not have a vested interest in the research sign a portion of the consent form indicating that, in his or her opinion, the patient was able to understand what was being asked. In cases where the patient has been judged to be incompetent (e.g. suffering from some severe psychiatric disorders, Alzheimer's disease, mental retardation, and the like), consent is gained from the legal guardian or next-of-kin, such as a spouse, child, or parent.

The other aspect of autonomy, in addition to the informed part, is *freedom to not participate in* or to *withdraw from* the study (hence, it is often referred to as 'free and informed consent'). This component of consent can be violated in ways which range from the blatantly obvious to the sublimely subtle. Since flagrant violations are easy to detect and are usually patently unethical, we will devote most of the discussion to the less obvious situations, where researchers may not even be aware of the fact that they are trespassing on dangerous territory.

Having Introductory Psychology students participate in studies as a requirement of the course or for extra marks has been a long, if not hallowed, tradition. (Indeed, as far back as 1946, McNemar referred to psychology as 'the science of the behavior of sophomores'.) However, this clearly obviates the freedom to withdraw, since to do so would result in a lower mark or perhaps even a failing grade. Many universities have banned this practice entirely, or allow the student to perform some other activity, such as writing a paper, as an alternative to serving as a research subject (American Psychological Association 1992).

A more subtle form of coercion may exist when a clinician recruits his or her patients to be research subjects. Some subjects may agree to participate because they are concerned that, if they do not, they will not receive the same level of care, despite assurances to the contrary. At one level, they are probably correct. Even if the clinician does not intend to withdraw services or to perform them in a more perfunctory manner, it is natural to assume that his or her attitude toward the patient may be affected by the latter's cooperation or refusal. Other patients may agree to participate out of a sense of gratitude; as a way of saying 'Thank you' for the treatment received. There is considerable debate whether this is a mild form of coercion, capitalizing on the patient's sense of obligation, or a very legitimate form of *quid pro quo*, allowing the patient to repay a perceived debt. Perhaps the safest course to take is for consent to be sought by a person not directly involved in the patient's care: a research assistant, teaching fellow, or by another, disinterested clinician.

The use of hospital or agency charts without the express permission of the patient is another area in which there is no consensus of opinion. The most stringent interpretation of the principle of consent is that in the absence of it, the researcher is prohibited from opening them. This would ban access to patient charts in such circumstances as: (a) gathering information to determine if those who refused to participate in a study differed in terms of demographic information from those who took part; (b) wanting to correlate test data with clinical information, such as the number of times a patient presented at the emergency room or at an outpatient clinic; or (c) even finding a group of patients who should later be approached to participate in a study (e.g. those with specific disorders, those who make frequent use of clinical services, or who have certain demographic characteristics).

It is obvious that this strict interpretation of consent would make some forms of research impossible, or at least extremely costly. A more liberal view is held by people such as Berg (1954), who states that, 'If the persons concerned are not harmed by the use of their records and their identities are not publicly revealed, there is no problem and their consent for the professional use of their records is not necessary' (p. 109). Most research ethics committees take an intermediate position, exemplified by the Ethical Principles of Research of the British Psychological Society (1977). It states that when there is any 'encroachment upon privacy', that the 'investigator should seek the opinion of experienced and disinterested colleagues', a rôle that is usually played now by the ethics committees of various institutions themselves. The Council for International Organizations of Medical Sciences (CIOMS 1993) adopts a similar position, explicitly stating that the review must be done by an ethical review committee, and further adds the stipulation that 'access ... must be supervised by a person who is fully aware of the confidentiality requirements' (p. 35).

This confidentiality of records continues after the data have been collected. The research guidelines of all psychological organizations have emphasized this point for both clinical and research findings (cf. Schuler 1982). Whenever possible, forms should be completed anonymously. However, this is not always feasible; it is sometimes necessary for the purposes of validity testing to link the results of the scale under development to other data, or, when test–retest reliability is being determined, to scores on the same measure completed at some later date. When this is the case, then (a) the data should be kept in a locked storage cabinet, to which only the researcher has access, and (b) the names should be removed and replaced by identification numbers as soon as possible.

Even when these precautions are taken, there may be circumstances (albeit admittedly rare) in which confidentiality cannot be maintained. In Example B, the data have been subpoenaed by a court. If the names have already been removed, and no key linking the names with the ID numbers exists, then there is no problem; the data are unretrievable in a form which can be linked to a specific individual. However, if the individual people are still identifiable for some of the reasons given above, then the test developer is legally obligated to provide the information, and can be cited for contempt of court if he or she does not. The rule of privileged communication does not apply in this case for a number of reasons. First, the researcher is most often not in a fiduciary or therapeutic relationship with the subject. Indeed, he or she may never have met the subject previously, and the contact was usually made at the researcher's initiative and for his or her purposes. Second, the rule is not universal, and rarely extends beyond lawyers and priests; psychologists, physicians, and other health providers are usually not protected.

Finally, there are situations where confidentiality must be violated by the researcher. These involve cases where the investigator believes that the subject is in imminent danger of harming him- or herself or other people. The person should be offered help and encouraged to seek professional advice. If the researcher feels that the danger is acute, and that the person is unwilling to be helped, then the 'duty to warn' supersedes the rules of confidentiality; this is called the Tarasoff rule, following the case of *Tarasoff v Regents of University of*

California in 1974. Even if the test is not yet validated, so that the researcher is not sure that a high score truly reflects emotional disturbance, it is often better to err on the side of intervening than simply dismissing the test as 'under development'.

In conclusion, the major issue confronting the scale developer is that of the autonomy of the subject. If the person is seen as an autonomous individual, who has the right to privacy and to not participate in the study irrespective of the difficulties this may pose for the researcher, then most problems should be avoidable.

References

American Educational Research Association, National Council on Measurement in Education (1955). *Technical recommendations for achievement tests*. American Psychological Association, Washington DC.

American Psychological Association (1954). *Technical recommendations for psychological tests and diagnostic techniques*. American Psychological Association, Washington DC.

American Psychological Association (1992). Ethical principles of psychologists and code of conduct. *American Psychologist*, **47**, 1597–1611.

Berg, I. A. (1954). The use of human subjects in psychological research. *American Psychologist*, **9**, 108–11.

British Psychological Society, Scientific Affairs Board (1977). Ethics of investigations with human subjects: A set of principles proposed by the Scientific Affairs Board. *Bulletin of the British Psychological Society*, **30**, 25–6.

Council for International Organizations of Medical Sciences (1993). *International ethical guidelines for biomedical research involving human subjects*. CIOMS, Geneva.

McNemar, Q. (1946). Opinion-attitude methodology. *Psychological Bulletin*, **43**, 289–374.

Medical Research Council of Canada. (1987). *Guidelines on research involving human subjects: 1987*. Medical Research Council of Canada, Ottawa, ON.

Novick, M. R. (1981). Federal guidelines and professional standards. *American Psychologist*, **36**, 1035–46.

Schuler, H. (1982). *Ethical problems in psychological research* (Trans. M. S. Woodruff and R. A. Wicklund). Academic Press, New York.

Shipley, T. (1977). Misinformed consent: An enigma in modern social science research. *Ethics in Science and Medicine*, **4**, 93–106.

Tarasoff *v* Regents of the University of California, 131 Cal. Rptr. 14, 551 P 2d 334 (1976).

Wilson, D. W. and Donnerstein, E. (1976). Legal and ethical aspects of nonreactive social psychological research. *American Psychologist*, **31**, 765–73.

Appendix A: Further reading

Chapter 1: Introduction

Colton, T. D. (1974). *Statistics in medicine*. Little Brown, Boston.
Freund, J. E. (1967). *Modern elementary statistics*. Prentice-Hall, Englewood Cliffs, NJ.
Huff, D. (1954). *How to lie with statistics*. W. W. Norton, New York.
Norman, G. R. and Streiner, D. L. (1987). *PDQ Statistics*. B. C. Decker, Toronto.
Norman, G. R. and Streiner, D. L. (1994). *Biostatistics: the bare essentials*. Mosby, St. Louis.

Chapter 2: Basic concepts

American Psychological Association (1985). *Standards for educational and psychological testing*. American Psychological Association, Washington.

Chapter 3: Developing the questions

Brislin, R. W. (1970). Back-translation for cross-cultural research. *Journal of Cross-Cultural Psychology*, **1**, 185–216.
Del Greco, L., Walop, W., and Eastridge, L. (1987). Questionnaire development: 3. Translation. *Canadian Medical Association Journal*, **136**, 817–18.
Oppenheim, A. N. (1966). *Questionnaire design and attitude measurement*. Heinemann, London.
Payne, S. L. (1951). *The art of asking questions*. Princeton University Press, Princeton, NJ.
Roid, G. H. and Haladyna, T. M. (1982). *A technology for test-item writing*. Academic Press, New York.
Sudman, S. and Bradburn, N. M. (1982). *Asking questions*. Jossey-Bass, San Francisco.

Chapter 4: Scaling approaches

Dunn-Rankin, P. (1983). *Scaling methods*. Erlbaum, Hillsdale, NJ.
Guilford, J. P. (1954). *Psychometric methods*. McGraw-Hill, New York.
TenBrick, T. D. (1974). *Evaluation: A practical guide for teachers*. McGraw-Hill, New York.

Chapter 5: Selecting the items

Anastasi, A. (1982). *Psychological testing* (5th edn), Chapter 8. Macmillan, New York.

Jackson, D. N. (1970). A sequential system for personality scale development. In *Current topics in clinical and community psychology* (ed. C. D. Spielberger), Vol. 2, pp. 61–96. Academic Press, New York.

Kornhauser, A. and Sheatsley, P. B. (1959). Questionnaire construction and interview procedure. In *Research methods in social relations* (eds. C. Selltiz, M. Jahoda, M. Deutsch, and S. W. Cook), rev. edn, pp. 546–87). Holt, Rinehart and Winston, New York.

Woodward, C. A. and Chambers, L. W. (1980). *Guide to questionnaire construction and question writing*. Canadian Public Health Association, Ottawa.

Chapter 6: Biases in question responses

Berg, I. A. (ed.) (1967). *Response set in personality assessment*. Aldine, Chicago.

Couch, A. and Keniston, K. (1960). Yeasayers and naysayers: Agreeing response set as a personality variable. *Journal of Abnormal and Social Psychology*, **60**, 151–74.

Edwards, A. L. (1957). *The social desirability variable in personality assessments and research*. Dryden, New York.

Thorndike, E. L. (1920). A constant error in psychological ratings. *Journal of Applied Psychology*, **4**, 25–9.

Warner, S. L. (1965). Randomized response: A survey technique for eliminating evasive answer bias. *Journal of the American Statistical Association*, **60**, 63–9.

Chapter 7: From items to scales

Nunnally, J. C., Jr. (1970). *Introduction to psychological measurement*, Chapter 8. McGraw-Hill, New York.

Chapter 8: Reliability

Anastasi, A. (1982). *Psychological testing* (5th edn), Chapter 5. Macmillan, New York.

Cronbach, L. J. (1984). *Essentials of psychological testing* (4th edn), Chapter 6. Harper and Row, New York.

Nunnally, J. C., Jr. (1970). *Introduction to psychological measurement*, Chapter 5. McGraw-Hill, New York.

Chapter 9: Generalizability theory

Brennan, R. L. (1983). *Elements of generalizability theory*. American College Testing Program, Iowa City.

Chapter 10: Validity

Anastasi, A. (1982). *Psychological testing* (5th edn). Chapters 6 and 7 Macmillan, New York.
Nunnally, J. C., Jr. (1970). *Introduction to psychological measurement*, Chapter 6. McGraw-Hill, New York.

Chapter 11: Measuring change

Nunnally, J. C., Jr. (1975). The study of change in evaluation research: Principles concerning measurement, experimental design, and analysis. In *Handbook of evaluation research* (eds. E. L. Struening and M. Guttentag), pp. 101–37. Sage, Beverly Hills.

Chapter 12: Latent-trait theories

Allen, M. J. and Yen, W. M. (1979). *Introduction to measurement theory*. Wadsworth, Belmont, CA.
Bejar, I. I. (1983). *Achievement testing*. Sage, Beverly Hills.
Crocker, L. and Algina, J. (1986). *Introduction to classical and modern test theory*. Holt, Rinehart, and Winston, New York.
Hambleton, R. K. (ed.) (1983). *Applications of item response theory*. Educational Research Institute of British Columbia, Vancouver.
Lord, F. M. (1980). *Application of item response theory to practical testing problems*. Erlbaum, Hillsdale, NJ.
Traub, R. E. and Wolfe, R. G. (1981). Latent trait theories and assessment of educational achievement. In *Review of research in education* 9, (ed. D. C. Berliner). American Educational Research Association, Washington DC.

Chapter 13: Methods of administration

Dillman, D. A. (1978). *Mail and telephone surveys: The total design method*. Wiley, New York.
Hyman, H. H., Cobb, W. J., Feldman, J. J., Hart, C. W., and Stember, C. H. (1954). *Interviewing in social research*. University of Chicago Press, Chicago.

Appendix B: Where to find tests

As mentioned in Chapter 3, a very useful place to find questions is to look at what others have done. Below is a partial listing of books and articles which are compendia of information about published and unpublished scales.

A. General

Backer, T. E. (1972). A reference guide for psychological measures. *Psychological Reports*, **31**, 751–68.
This article is an inventory of people, publications, and projects which may help in locating tests or information about them. It does not list any tests itself, only very useful information regarding finding them.

Behavioral Measurement Database Services. *Health and psychosocial instruments database* (HAPI). BRS Retrieval Service.
This is an on-line, computerized database, similar to MEDLINE or PsychInfo, containing over 6000 documents (as of August 1992) which provides information on various instruments. It covers health, social sciences, organizational behaviour, and human resources. Coverage is comprehensive from 1985 to the present, with many earlier measures included on a more haphazard basis. At the current time, the cost to use it is $55 US, or $88 Canadian per hour.

The mental measurements yearbooks. Buros Institute of Mental Measurements, Lincoln.
The first eight editions of the *MMY* were edited by Oscar Buros, and the set is often referred to as 'Buros'. After his death, J. V. Mitchell took over editorship of this excellent series. Only published tests are listed, and most are reviewed by two or more experts in the field. The articles also include a fairly comprehensive list of published articles and dissertations about the instruments. The yearbooks, which are not published annually, are cumulative: tests reviewed in one edition are not necessarily reviewed in subsequent ones.
The same group has also brought out more focused indices: *Reading tests and reviews*, *Tests in print*, and *Personality tests*. The latter two volumes do not have reviews, but the reader is directed back to the *MMY*.

Cattell, R. G. and Warburton, F. (1967). *Objective personality and motivation tests*. University of Illinois Press, Urbana, IL.
Although dated now, this book lists over 600 personality tests for adults and children. The psychometric properties of each are given, along with some sample test items.

Keyser, D. J. and Sweetland, R. C. *Test critiques*. Test Corporation of America, Kansas City, MO.
As of 1993, this series consists of nine volumes of critical evaluations of published tests. Unlike the *MMY*, there is only one review per test, and the reference list is representative rather than exhaustive. However, the reviews tend to be considerably longer and more detailed, and follow a common format: introduction, practical applications and uses, technical aspects, and critique.

Sweetland, R. C. and Keyser, D. J. (1986). *Tests: A comprehensive reference for assessments in psychology, education, and business* (2nd edn). Test Corporation of America, Kansas City, MO.
The main volume and the *Supplement* are similar to *Tests in print*. A description is given of over 3000 published tests: purpose, format, description, appropriate population, approximate time to complete them, and where to order.

Directory of unpublished experimental mental measures. Hume Sciences Press, New York.
One of the few comprehensive sources of scales which have appeared in journals but have not been published. Volume 1 (1974) was edited by B. A. Goldman and J. L. Saunders; Volumes 2 (1978) and 3 (1982) by Goldman and J. C. Busch; and Volume 4 (1985) by Goldman and W. L. Osborne. Each test is described and one or two key articles cited. There are no reviews.

B. Social and attitudinal scales

Bearden, W. O., Netemeyer, R. G., and Mobley, M. F. (1993). *Handbook of marketing scales*. Sage, Newbury Park.
The focus of the book is on consumer behaviour and marketing research. However, it also covers tests of individual traits which may have a rôle in such behaviours, such as values, susceptibility to peer pressure, materialism, and the like. Over 100 scales are covered; for each, there is a brief review of the psychometric properties, as well as a copy of the tool itself.

Bonjean, C. M., Hill, R. J., and McLemore, S. D. (1967). *Sociological measurement*. Chandler, San Francisco.
Lists every scale used in four sociology journals between 1954 and 1965. Over 2000 measures are listed, with comprehensive references.

Heitzman, C. A. and Kaplan, R. M. (1988). Assessment of methods for measuring social support. *Health Psychology*, **7**, 75–109.
This is a critical review of 24 of the more widely used social support scales. The scales themselves are not given, but the assessments of them are excellent.

Miller, D. C. (1970). *Handbook of research design and social measurement* (2nd edn). McKay, New York.
Provides lists and examples of 36 sociometric scales in the areas of social status, group structure and dynamics, morale, job satisfaction, and the like.

Price, J. M. and Mueller, C. W. (1986). *Handbook of organizational measures*. Pitman, Marshfield, MA.
Although oriented toward people in businesses, this book also covers such topics as autonomy, communication, and satisfaction. There are a total of 30 areas, with usually one test per area reviewed. Representative items are given for some of the scales.

Robinson, J. P., Athanasiou, R., and Head, K. B. (1969). *Measures of occupational attitudes and occupational characteristics*. Institute of Social Research, Ann Arbor.
Robinson, J. P., Rusk, J. G., and Head, K. B. (1968). *Measures of political attitude*. Institute of Social Research, Ann Arbor.

Robinson, J. P. and Shaver, P. R. (1969). *Measures of social psychological attitudes*. Institute of Social Research, Ann Arbor.
These three volumes from the ISR provide the actual items comprising the various scales. Each volume lists between 30 and 90 scales, with a short critique of each.

Shaw, M. E. and Wright, J. M. (1967). *Scales for the measurement of attitudes*. Institute of Social Research, Ann Arbor.
176 scales are described and listed, covering such areas as international and social issues, social practices and problems, political and religious attitudes, and so forth.

C. Personality

Chéné, H. (1986). *Index des variables mesurées par les tests de personalité* (2nd edn). Les Presses de l'Université Laval, Laval Quebec.
Brief, non-evaluative descriptions of primarily published tests. In French.

Chun, K-T., Cobb, S., and French, J. R. P., Jr. (1975). *Measures for psychological assessment: A guide to 3,000 original sources and their applications*. Institute of Social Research, Ann Arbor.
A listing of 3000 articles which have used various psychological tests, keyed back to the original scales.

Lake, D. G., Miles, M., and Earle, R. (1973). *Measuring human behavior*. Teachers College Press, New York.
This book gives psychometric data on 84 tests in the areas of personal attributes, interpersonal and organizational relationships, and the like. The tests themselves are not given.

D. Child and family

Center for the Study of Evaluation. (1970). *Elementary school test evaluations*. Author, Los Angeles.
Center for the Study of Evaluation. (1971). *Preschool/kindergarten test evaluations*. Author, Los Angeles.
These two volumes are designed for both professionals and school administrators. Critical evaluations are provided for tests focussed on educational objectives.

Johnson, O. G. (1976). *Tests and measurements in child development: Handbooks I and II*. Jossey-Bass, San Francisco.
This is an update of Johnson and Bommarito's earlier book, which was subtitled simply, *A handbook*. The two volumes now cover 1200 non-commercial tests which are appropriate for those under 19 years of age. A wide variety of areas are covered, and the psychometric properties of each test are described.

Levy, P. and Goldstein, H. (eds). *Tests in education: A book of critical reviews*. Academic Press, London.
Similar in design and intent to the *MMY* and *Test critiques*, this volume is oriented toward published tests available in England, which do not need to be administered by a psychologist, and which cover children from nursery school through secondary school.

Orvaschel, H., Sholomskas, D., and Weissman, M. M. (1980). *The assessment of psychopathology and behavioral problems in children: A review of scales suitable for epidemiological and clinical research (1967-1979).* NIMH, Rockville, MD.

Orvaschel, H. and Walsh, G. (1984). *The assessment of adaptive functioning in children: A review of existing measures suitable for epidemiological and clinical services research.* NIMH, Rockville, MD.

These two monographs list and critique unpublished scales which can be used with children under the age of 18.

Straus, M. A. and Brown, B. W. (1978). *Family measurement techniques: Abstracts of published instruments, 1935–1974* (revised edn). University of Minnesota Press, Minneapolis.

This book consists of descriptions of 813 family behaviour measures, culled from journals in psychology, education, and sociology, and covering husband–wife interactions, parent–child and sibling interactions, and sex and premarital relations. Each scale is described, with a few representative items given.

Walker, D. K. (1973). *Socioemotional measures for preschool and kindergarten children.* Jossey-Bass, San Francisco.

This covers published and unpublished, copyrighted and freely available tests for children between the ages of 3 and 6. There are psychometric data given for 143 instruments.

E. Health

Bowling, A. (1991). *Measuring health: A review of quality of life measurement scales.* Open University Press, Philadelphia.

The book reviews scales in five areas: functional ability, health status, psychological well-being, social networks and support, and life satisfaction and morale. Each test is described and evaluated, and representative items given for each.

Comrey, A. L., Backer, T. E., and Glaser, E. M. (1973). *A sourcebook for mental health measures.* Human Interaction Research Institute, Los Angeles.

Consists of over 1000 abstracts of mental health measures. Some reliability and validity data are given for each scale; the scales themselves are not reproduced.

Corcoran, K. and Fischer, J. (1987). *Measures for clinical practice.* The Free Press, New York.

This book covers 127 scales: 92 for adults, 19 for children, and 16 for couples and families. For each scale, there are brief notes about its purpose, norms, scoring, reliability, and validity. The entire scale is also reprinted, although the scoring key is not. An excellent sourcebook for scales and items.

Hersen, M. and Bellack, A. S. (eds.) (1988). *Dictionary of behavioral assessment techniques.* Pergamon, New York.

The book covers many different techniques to measure attributes such as anxiety, assertiveness, beliefs, and skills. Some of the techniques are scales, while others are structured tasks or even pieces of electronic equipment. The psychometric characteristics of each procedure are given, but the scales themselves are not reproduced.

McDowell, I. and Newell, C. (1987). *Measuring health: A guide to rating scales and questionnaires*. Oxford University Press, Oxford.
This book reviews 50 scales in the areas of physical disability, psychological well-being, social health, pain, and quality of life. Each scale is described in detail, often with example questions, and its reliability and validity are reviewed. An excellent guide.

Reader, L. G. Ramacher, L., and Gorelnik, S. (1976). *Handbook of scales and indices of health behavior*. Goodyear Publishing, Pacific Palisades, CA.
For each test within the areas of health behaviour, health status, and utilization, psychometric data are presented, as well as copies of the scales themselves.

Stewart, A. L. and Ware, J. E. (eds.) (1992). *Measuring functioning and well-being*. Duke University Press, Durham, NC.
This book focuses on the tests used in a very large study, the Medical Outcome Study. Within this limited scope, it provides useful information on some indices for social and role functioning, psychological distress, pain, sleep, and the like.

Wilkin, D., Hallam, L., and Doggett, M. A. (1992). *Measures of need and outcome for primary health care*. Oxford University Press, Oxford.
This book covers tests in seven areas: functioning, mental health and illness, social support, patient satisfaction, disease-specific questionnaires, multi-dimensional tests, and miscellaneous. A number of tests in each area are reviewed. For copyrighted ones, a representative item is presented; for others, the whole test is shown.

F. Gerontology

Mangen, D. J. and Peterson, W. A. (eds.) *Research instruments in social gerontology*. University of Minnesota Press, Minneapolis.
There are three volumes in this series. Volume 1 (1982) is subtitled *Clinical and social psychology*, Volume 2 (1982) is called *Social roles and social participation*, and Volume 3 (1984) covers *Health, program evaluation, and demography*. Each chapter reviews the scales in one area, giving a description of them, brief comments on reliability and validity, and a copy of the scales themselves.

G. Nursing

Frank-Stromborg, M. (ed.) (1988). *Instruments for clinical nursing research*. Appleton & Lange, Norwalk, CN.
Each of the book's 24 chapters covers a different functional area or clinical problem, such as quality of life, sleep, dyspnoea, pain, or spirituality. Numerous scales are briefly mentioned within each chapter, and most get only one or two paragraphs. A good source of tests, but weak on evaluation.

Waltz, C. F. and Strickland, O. L. (eds.) (1988). *Measurement of nursing outcomes: Vol. I. Measuring client outcomes*. Springer, New York.
Strickland, O. L., and Waltz, C. F. (eds.) (1988). *Measurement of nursing outcomes: Vol. II. Measuring nursing performance: Practice, education, and research*. Springer, New York.

The first volume consists of 25 chapters, covering such topics as illness-oriented measures, measuring wellness, quality of care, and factors in community based care. Each chapter focuses on and reproduces usually one or two measures, with some psychometric data. The second volume looks at measuring professionalism, clinical performance, and educational outcomes, using a similar format.

Ward, M. J. and Fetler, M. E. (1979). *Instruments for use in nursing education research.* Western Interstate Commission for Higher Education, Boulder, CO.

A wide variety of instruments is presented, ranging from achievement tests of nursing knowledge to attitudes toward nursing and toward various patient groups, learning styles, and so on. Each test is shown in full, with some discussion of its psychometric properties.

Author Index

Subject Index